INSTANT NURSING ASSESSMENT:

$\mathscr{N}$eurologic

▽   ▽   ▽   ▽   .▽   ▽   ▽

Delmar Publishers' Online Services

To access Delmar on the World Wide Web, point your browser to:

http://www.delmar.com/delmar.html

To access through Gopher:

gopher://gopher.delmar.com

(Delmar Online is part of "thomson.com," an Internet site with information on more than 30 publishers of the International Thomson Publishing organization.)

For more information on our products and services:

email: info@delmar.com or call 800-347-7707

INSTANT NURSING ASSESSMENT:

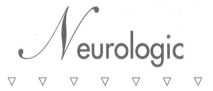

$\mathscr{N}$eurologic

▽ ▽ ▽ ▽ ▽ ▽ ▽

Judith A. Mauro, RN, BS, MA, CNA
Nurse Manager
St. Peter's Medical Center
New Brunswick, New Jersey

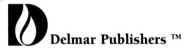 **Delmar Publishers** ™

I(T)P™ An International Thomson Publishing Company

Albany • Bonn • Boston • Cincinnati • Detroit • London • Madrid
Melbourne • Mexico City • New York • Pacific Grove • Paris • San Francisco
Singapore • Tokyo • Toronto • Washington

$\mathcal{S}$TAFF

Team Leader:
DIANE McOSCAR

Sponsoring Editors:
PATRICIA CASEY
BILL BURGOWER

Developed for Delmar Publishers by:
JENNINGS & KEEFE Media Development, Corte Madera, CA

Concept, Editorial, and Design Management:
THE WILLIAMS COMPANY, LTD., Collegeville, PA

Project Coordinator:
KATHLEEN LUCZAK

Editorial Administrator:
GABRIEL DAVIS

Production Editor:
BARBARA HODGSON

Manuscript written by:
TRACI A. GINNONA

Text Design:
KM DESIGN GROUP

For information, address:
Delmar Publishers
3 Columbia Circle
Box 15015
Albany, NY 12212-5015

International Thomson Publishing Europe
Berkshire House 168-173
High Holborn
London, WC1V7AA
England

Thomas Nelson Australia
102 Dodds Street
South Melbourne, 3205
Victoria, Australia

Nelson Canada
1120 Birchmount Road
Scarborough, Ontario
Canada M1K 5G4

International Thomson Editores
Campos Eliseos 385, Piso 7
Col Polanco
11560 Mexico D F Mexico

International Thomson Publishing GmbH
Königswinterer Strasse 418
53227 Bonn
Germany

International Thomson Publishing Asia
221 Henderson Road
#05-10 Henderson Building
Singapore 0315

International Thomson Publishing Japan
Hirakawacho Kyowa Building, 3F
2-2-1 Hirakawacho
Chiyoda-ku, Tokyo 102
Japan

Printed in the United States of America

Published simultaneously in Canada

by Nelson Canada, a division of The Thomson Corporation.

1 2 3 4 5 6 7 8 9 10 XXX 00 99 98 97 96 95

Library of Congress Cataloging-in-Publication Data
Mauro, Judith A., 1956-
    Instant nursing assessment: neurologic/Judith A. Mauro.
        p. cm. — (Instant nursing assessment)
    Includes bibliographical references and index.
    ISBN 0-8273-7103-9
        1. Neurological nursing. 2. Nursing assessment. I. Title. II. Series.
        [DNLM: 1. Nervous System Diseases—nursing. 2.Nervous System Diseases—diagnosis—nurses' instruction. 3. Nursing Assessment—methods. WY 160.5 M457i 1995]
    RC350.5.M38 1995
    610.73'68—dc20
    DNLM/DLC
    for Library of Congress   95-24076
                                                                CIP

$\mathcal{T}$ITLES IN THIS SERIES:

Suzanne K. Marnocha, RN, MSN, CCRN
Assistant Professor, College of Nursing
University of Wisconsin
Oshkosh, Wisconsin

Linda Moody, RN, FAAN, Ph.D.
Professor, Director of Research and Chair,
Gerontology Nursing
College of Nursing
University of South Florida
Tampa, Florida

Patricia A. O'Neill, RN, CCRN, MSN
Instructor, DeAnza College School of Nursing
Cupertino, California

Virgil Parsons, RN, DNSc, Ph.D.
Professor, School of Nursing
San Jose State University
San Jose, California

Elaine Rooney, MSN
Assistant Professor of Nursing, Nursing Department
University of Pittsburgh at Bradford
Bradford, Pennsylvania

Barbara Shafner, RN, Ph.D.
Associate Professor, Department of Nursing
Otterbein College
Westerville, Ohio

Elaine Souder, RN, Ph.D.
Associate Professor, College of Nursing
University of Arkansas for Medical Sciences
Little Rock, Arkansas

Mary Tittle, RN, Ph.D.
Associate Professor, College of Nursing
University of South Florida
Tampa, Florida

Peggy L. Wros, RN, Ph.D.
Assistant Professor of Nursing
Linfield College School of Nursing
Portland, Oregon

CONTENTS

$\mathscr{N}$OTICE TO THE READER

The publisher, editors, advisors, and reviewers do not warrant or guarantee any of the products described herein nor have they performed any independent analysis in connection with any of the product information contained herein. The publisher, editors, advisors, and reviewers do not assume, and each expressly disclaims, any obligation to obtain and include information other than that provided to them by the manufacturer.

The reader is expressly warned to consider and adopt all safety precautions that might be indicated by the activities described herein and to avoid all potential hazards. By following the instructions contained herein, the reader willingly assumes all risks in connection with such instructions.

The publisher, editors, advisors, and reviewers make no representations or warranties of any kind, including but not limited to the warranties of fitness for particular purpose or merchantability, nor are any such representations implied with respect to the material set forth herein, and the publisher, editors, advisors, and reviewers take no responsibility with respect to such material. The publisher, editors, advisors, and reviewers shall not be liable for any special, consequential, or exemplary damages resulting, in whole or in part, from readers' use of, or reliance upon, this material.

A conscientious effort has been made to ensure that the drug information and recommended dosages in this book are accurate and in accord with accepted standards at the time of publication. However, pharmacology is a rapidly changing science, so readers are advised, before administering any drug, to check the package insert provided by the manufacturer for the recommended dose, for contraindications for administration, and for added warnings and precautions. This recommendation is especially important for new, infrequently used, or highly toxic drugs.

CPR standards are subject to frequent change due to ongoing research. The American Heart Association can verify changing CPR standards when applicable. Recommended Schedules for Immunization are also subject to frequent change. The American Academy of Pediatrics, Committee on Infectious Diseases can verify changing recommendations.

FOREWORD

As quality and cost-effectiveness continue to drive rapid change within the health care system, you must respond quickly and surely— whether you are a student, a novice, or an expert. This *Instant Assessment Series*—and its companion *Nursing Interventions Series*— will help you do that by providing a great deal of nursing information in short, easy-to-read columns, charts, and boxes. This convenient presentation will support you as you practice your science and art and apply the nursing process. I hope you'll come to look on these books as providing "an experienced nurse in your pocket."

The *Instant Assessment Series* offers immediate, relevant clinical information on the most important aspects of patient assessment. The *Nursing Interventions Series* is a handy source for appropriate step-by-step nursing actions to ensure quality care and meet the fast-paced challenges of today's nursing profession. Because more nurses will be working in out-patient settings as we move into the 21st century, these series include helpful information about ambulatory patients.

These books contain several helpful special features, including nurse alerts to warn you quickly about critical assessment findings, nursing diagnoses charts that include interventions and rationales along with collaborative management to help you work with your health care colleagues, patient teaching tips, and the latest nursing research findings.

Each title in the *Instant Assessment Series* begins with a review of general health assessment tools and techniques and then expands to cover a different body system, such as cardiovascular, or a special group of patients, such as pediatric or geriatric. This focused approach allows each book to provide extensive information—but in a quick reference format—to help you grow and excel in your specialty.

Both medical and nursing diagnoses are included to help you adapt to emerging critical pathways, care mapping, and decision trees. All these new guidelines help decrease length of stay and increase quality of care—all current health care imperatives.

I'm confident that each small but powerful volume will prove indispensable in your nursing practice. Each book is formatted to help you quickly connect your assessment findings with the patient's pathophysiology—a cognitive connection that will further help you plan nursing interventions, both independent and collaborative, to care for your patients skillfully and completely. With the help and guidance provided by the books in this series, you will be able to thrive—and survive—in these changing times.

— Helene K. Nawrocki, RN, MSN, CNA
Executive Vice President
The Center for Nursing Excellence
Newtown, Pennsylvania
Adjunct Faculty, La Salle University
Philadelphia, Pennsylvania

$\mathcal{C}$hapter 1. Health History

▽   ▽   ▽   ▽   ▽   ▽   ▽

$\mathcal{I}$NTRODUCTION

SEE TEXT PAGES

When taking a health history, collect critical subjective data about the patient. In addition to collecting clues about existing or possible health problems, you are also drawing a road map for future patient interactions. To make this map as useful as possible, gather information about the patient's physical condition and symptoms and explore the patient's psychological, cultural, and psychosocial environment as it pertains to his or her health issues.

$\mathcal{B}$EGINNING CONSIDERATIONS

Collecting vital information about the patient can be a daunting task. Patients are often nervous and apprehensive. They may also feel awkward or embarrassed about sharing their problems and concerns, particularly if they've never seen you before. You may even feel some anxiety about the prospective interview.

You can do several things to ease the situation:
• Create a comfortable physical environment.
• Learn interviewing techniques that will put the patient at ease.

$\mathcal{T}$HE EXTERNAL ENVIRONMENT

The external environment is the place where you meet with the patient to collect the health history.

Do the following to help the patient feel at ease:
• Conduct the interview in a quiet, private area.
• Set the thermostat at a comfortable level.
• Make sure the lighting is adequate.
• Avoid interruptions.
• Remove objects that might upset or distract the patient.
• Position yourself and the patient as equals by:
  - Sitting in comfortable chairs at eye level. Standing implies that you are more powerful.
  - Not interviewing the patient from behind a desk or table.

- Maintain an appropriate distance between you and the patient. Be sensitive to cultural differences and the need for personal space.

Communicating with Your Patient

Successful communication requires good interpersonal skills that place the patient at ease. To do so, use the techniques suggested by the acronym DEAR:

- Demonstrate acceptance
- Empathize openly
- Affirm
- Recognize

The best way to show a patient that you accept what he or she is saying is to listen. People know that you are listening when you make comments like "I see what you are saying" or simply, "I understand." When you nod your head yes and make eye contact, you also show that you are attentive and accepting of what you hear. Acceptance is not the same as believing the patient's statements are right or wrong.

Empathy is the uniquely human ability to put yourself in someone else's shoes, to show that you can relate to his or her feelings. You show empathy when you say such things as "That must have made you sad/frightened/happy/relieved."

When you affirm and recognize, you are putting acceptance and empathy to work. Affirmation is the act of acknowledging what the patient is telling you.

Recognition is listening well and attentively, thus showing the patient by what you say and how you say it that you hear him or her. It can be as simple as nodding yes or saying "Please continue."

Some patients will come to you with as many concerns about the treatment process and environment as about their health. Reassure them that all communication is confidential and that you cannot legally reveal anything beyond the confines of the health care team without the patient's consent.

ℰNSURING A SUCCESSFUL INTERVIEW

Sometimes patients are so apprehensive or have had such negative health care experiences that they are hostile. To best handle such a patient, follow these guidelines:

- Remain calm.
- Never argue with the patient.
- Affirm and recognize his or her feelings using simple sentences.
- Reschedule the interview if the patient's hostility persists.
- If you feel physically intimidated by the patient, call for assistance.

A second factor that can skew the results of your interview is a cultural or ethnic difference between you and the patient. Differences between cultures can be subtle. For example, in the United States, most people consider it rude not to make eye contact. Culturally, the absence of eye contact suggests disinterest or dishonesty. In many other cultures, it is considered extremely rude to make eye contact with elders or authority figures, or eye contact is not made between unrelated members of the opposite sex.

While it is important to be sensitive to cultural differences, try not to go to the other extreme and resort to stereotyping. Each of us is a unique individual regardless of our culture. No one perfectly embodies all the characteristics of a culture.

Sometimes we use the term "ethnic group" to refer to a group that shares a common culture. At other times we use the same term to refer to a group that shares a common biological origin. On still other occasions we use the term to refer to a group that shares a common national origin. Beware of making judgments about a patient's behavior based on biological ethnicity. Skin color is not a good predictor of cultural affiliation. People who are "American" come in all sizes, shapes, and colors.

Pay attention to how culture and individual character affect the patient's lifestyle, fears and hopes about his or her health, and feelings about treatment. This can be an exciting journey for both of you.

THE INTERVIEW: YOUR ROLE

The interview involves two persons—you and the patient—and is really the sum of what both of you bring to it. You, however, are the authority figure, and most patients will expect you to set the tone and direction of the interview. Your goal is to help the patient become a willing participant in his or her own care—to actively assist in discovering solutions to problems he or she may experience. The more you know about successful interviewing techniques, the more likely you are to be at ease with the patient. Remember: These techniques are general guidelines. You are the best judge of what is most effective in any given situation.

Like a college essay, the interview can be broken into three parts: the introduction, the main body (the interview), and the conclusion (parting with the patient).

THE INTRODUCTION

The introductory phase of the interview sets the tone for the rest of the assessment. It's also where you begin to build a rapport with the patient.
- Always start the interview by introducing yourself and giving the patient some background on your place in the organization. It may help to shake hands. Always ask the patient how he or she likes to be addressed.
- Take a little time to get to know the patient by talking informally before you begin the interview process.

NURSE ALERT:
Make sure the patient speaks fluent English. If not, you may want to postpone the interview until you can obtain an interpreter.

- Explain how long the interview will take.
- Describe the interview process and ask the patient for questions.
- If you need to take notes to remember information, tell the patient you will be doing so in order to listen more attentively.

THE INTERVIEW

The main body of the interview is where you collect the information you need for the patient's treatment and care. Provide a road map. Begin the interview process by asking general questions. Ask the patient why he or she came in for today's visit. During the interview, help the patient by asking questions such as "Is there anything else you're worried about?"

Repeat important points the patient makes. You can make a comment such as "You just said that your pain occurs early in the morning. Let's explore that for a second."

Another way to draw the road map is to interpret what the patient has said and done. You could say, "It sounds like whenever you are short of breath, something has happened to make you anxious." Clarify the patient's statement as much as possible.

In other situations, the patient may have trouble verbalizing his or her concerns. In this case, a response like "It seems to me that you are concerned about..." shows that you will do whatever is necessary to help the patient communicate more clearly.

Finally, you can help the patient be clear by summarizing major points with statements such as "So far, we've talked about...I think we are ready to go on to talk about...."

Give the patient time to think about what he or she needs to say. This shows that you respect the patient's thought process. Use silence to focus on the patient's nonverbal behavior.

Be an observer. Be aware of the patient's unspoken behavior. When appropriate, use these observations for clarification and to heighten the patient's awareness. Simple observations such as "It appears that that must have been a painful experience" often open new avenues for exploration and discovery.

Affirm the patient's role in the interview as a participant. For example, ask the patient to offer strategies for dealing with his or her health care issues.

Sometimes patients may make statements or have expectations that are unrealistic. Respond by pointing out the obvious—"You told me your side doesn't bother you, but you wince every time I touch it." Or you might say, "You'll feel much better after treatment, but you won't be able to go back to long-distance running."

It is very important that the patient remain grounded. Comments such as "You look worried," "You seem tense," and "You sound more relaxed" affirm the patient's feelings.

You can empower patients to be willing participants in the interview process by openly sharing whatever information and facts you have about their health care and the decisions involved in it. Clearly explain patient care and how the health care system works.

AVOIDING PITFALLS

Just as there are good techniques for interviewing, there are techniques to avoid because they increase tension and reduce communication between you and the patient.

- Justification. When you ask patients how or why something happened, you are implying that they need to explain or defend their behavior. You can also make a patient feel you expect an explanation when you ask leading questions. A leading question always implies that there is a single "right" answer. For example, "You don't eat a lot of fried foods, do you?" is likely to get a no from even the most dedicated french-fry eater.
- Too persistent. There is an old saying about not beating a dead horse that applies to interviews. If you don't get the desired information after a couple of tries, move on.
- The wrong tone. Be careful to gear your discussion to the patient's ability to understand it. On the one hand, don't overwhelm the patient with technical terms and medical jargon. On the other hand, don't talk down to the patient.

Pay attention to how the patient prefers to be addressed. For example, an older woman may find it patronizing and rude if you address her by her first name.

If you are talking about death, use statements such as "he died," not "he's gone to his reward." Pay attention to such euphemisms when used by the patient. They are a way to avoid real feelings, and we most often resort to them when talking about subjects that make us feel anxious or frightened.

Be personable but not personal. If you begin to share your own experiences or provide advice, you are likely to make the patient feel like a nonparticipant in the health care process.

The patient who asks for advice is demonstrating respect and trust. You can repay that with responses such as "Even if I were in the exact same situation as you, I might not want to do the same thing. What do you think is best for you?"

While touch can be comforting to a patient, too much of it can feel inappropriate. Likewise, be aware of becoming too impersonal. When you assume the posture of an authority figure, you create distance between you and the patient. To say, "I'm the nurse and I know best," even when a patient is clearly doing something destructive like smoking, implies that the patient is inferior to you.

Another way to be too impersonal is to use impersonal language. It is the difference between "That wasn't very clear" and "I don't understand." The first statement removes you from the equation. Also, consider the following:

- Losing touch with reality. Making statements such as "It will all be OK," "Don't worry, you'll be fine," or "Life goes on" may make you feel better, but they don't make the patient feel better. Rather, the patient is likely to feel that you don't care about the impact of his or her illness or that you cannot be trusted to tell the truth.
- Interrupting. If you interrupt the patient or change the subject, you are likely to make the patient feel that you are impatient. The same is true of drawing conclusions too quickly. When you draw all the conclusions, the patient is likely to withhold information or tell you what he or she thinks you want to hear.
- Inappropriate emotion. Inappropriate responses to what the patient says include the following:
  - Don't overly praise the response. If, for example, our french-fry eater said no to your leading question about fried foods and you responded with "That's fantastic. It's great that you're so disciplined," you're not likely to find out what his diet and exercise patterns really are.
  - Don't show disapproval or anger.
  - Don't take the patient too literally. If a patient says he is not afraid of needles but pulls his arm away, shuts his eyes, and grits his teeth, he is clearly apprehensive about injections. It's important that you base your response as much on what the patient does as what the patient says.

*P*ARTING WITH THE PATIENT

How you close the interview is as important as how you open and conduct it. Ask the patient if he or she has any other questions or comments and how he or she feels about the treatment decisions. Summarize the information collected in the interview and any decisions that have been made about future treatment. Make sure you and the patient understand this in the same way.

*N*ONVERBAL CUES

Not all communication is spoken. In fact, the majority of communication is nonverbal. You can learn to send nonverbal messages to your patient that emphasize the qualities of DEAR discussed earlier in this chapter.

- Appearance. Be appropriately professional. Avoid dressing in a way that makes the patient uncomfortable.
- Posture. Be relaxed. Keep your arms uncrossed to convey openness. Direct your body toward your patient. Don't slouch.
- Gestures. Occasionally, you can use your hands to encourage conversation. Touch the patient's arm for comfort. Never point at the patient, clench your fist, or drum your fingers. Avoid looking at your watch. Never touch the patient in a way that he or she may find inappropriate.
- Facial expression. Try to look actively interested. Smile and show concern when appropriate. Avoid yawning, which expresses boredom. Try not to frown, grimace, or chew on your lip or cheek. Maintain appropriate eye contact.
- Speech. Keep your voice moderate. Raise it only if the patient has trouble hearing. Watch your tone of voice with patients who speak English as a second language. We all have a tendency to yell when trying to make ourselves understood. Make sure you are not speaking too quickly or too slowly.

*T*AKING THE HEALTH HISTORY: PRELIMINARY MATERIAL

Having laid out the structure of the interview, it is now time to get down to specifics. Each institution has its own form. Be complete in filling out the form specific to your institution. The table that follows lists initial information you should obtain from your patient.

NURSE ALERT:
If the patient is feeling ill, begin by collecting the relevant information about his or her illness. Collect other information afterward or reschedule the patient. Don't tax the patient's energy with the interview.

HEALTH HISTORY CHECKLIST

AREA TO COVER	SPECIFIC QUESTIONS
Biographical information	Use the form your institution provides.
Allergies	Are you allergic to any: • medications (include reaction) • foods (include reaction) • environmental agents (include reaction)
Medication	What medications (including dosages) do you take on a regular basis? Include both prescription and over-the-counter medications.
Childhood illnesses	Have you had measles, mumps, rubella, chicken pox, pertussis, strep throat, rheumatic fever, scarlet fever, poliomyelitis?
Accidents or injuries	Describe and include dates of any accidents or injuries you've had.
Chronic illnesses	Do you have diabetes, hypertension, heart disease, sickle cell anemia, cancer, AIDS, seizure disorder?

HEALTH HISTORY CHECKLIST *(CONTINUED)*

AREA TO COVER	SPECIFIC QUESTIONS
Hospitalizations	Describe, including dates and diagnoses, any hospitalizations.
Surgical procedures	Describe, with dates and diagnoses, any operations.
Obstetric	How many times have you been pregnant? How many full-term pregnancies have you had? Have you had any abortions?
Immunizations	Did you receive the complete battery of childhood immunizations? What is the date of your most recent tetanus shot, hepatitis B vaccine, tuberculin skin test, flu shot?
Last examination	When were your most recent physical, dental, and eye examinations; hearing test; ECG; and chest X-ray performed?

PHYSIOLOGICAL ASSESSMENT: GENERAL

The following table lists general physiological questions to ask the patient. If the patient is not feeling well, go on to the table titled "Current Complaint." If possible, also cover the family history information listed in the "Family Environment" table.

AREA TO COVER	SPECIFIC QUESTIONS
Present health status	Have you had any recent weight gain or loss? Do you know the cause? Do you experience any of the following? • fatigue, weakness, or malaise • difficulty in carrying out daily activities • fever or chills • sweats or night sweats • frequent colds or other infections Are you able to exercise?
Skin	Do you have a history of any of the following: • eczema, psoriasis, or hives • changes in pigment • changes in any moles • overly dry skin • overly moist skin • excessive bruising • pruritus • rashes • lesions • reaction to heat or cold • itching • sun exposure and amount Describe the location of any growths, moles, tumors, warts, or other skin abnormalities.

PHYSIOLOGICAL ASSESSMENT: GENERAL *(CONTINUED)*

AREA TO COVER	SPECIFIC QUESTIONS
Hair	Describe any recent hair loss, change in hair texture, or change in hair characteristics. How often do you shampoo your hair? Is your hair color-treated or permed? How often do you have this done?
Nails	Have you experienced any of the following: • changes in nail color • changes in nail texture • occurrences of nail splitting, cracking, or breaking • changes in nail shape
Head and neck	Have you experienced any of the following: • frequent or severe headaches • dizziness • pain or stiffness • a head injury • abnormal range of motion • surgery • enlarged glands • vertigo • lumps, bumps, or scars
Eyes	Have you been troubled by any of the following? • eye infections or trauma • eye pain • redness or swelling • change in vision

PHYSIOLOGICAL ASSESSMENT: GENERAL *(CONTINUED)*

AREA TO COVER	SPECIFIC QUESTIONS
Eyes *(continued)*	Have you been troubled by any of the following? • eye infections or trauma • eye pain • redness or swelling • change in vision • spots or other disturbances of the visual field • twitching or other sensations • strabisimus or amblyopia • itching, tearing, or discharge • double vision • glaucoma • cataracts • blurred vision, blind spots, or decreased visual acuity Do you wear glasses? Do you have a history of retinal detachment? When did you last have a glaucoma test and what was the result?
Ears	Have you experienced any of the following? • ear infections or earaches (include dates and frequency) • hearing loss • tinnitus (ringing or crackling) • exposure to environmental noise • discharge from the ear—color, frequency, and amount • vertigo • unusual sensitivity to noise • sensation of fullness in the ears When did you last have an ear examination? What was the result? What impact does your hearing loss have on your daily activities? How do you clean your ears?

PHYSIOLOGICAL ASSESSMENT: GENERAL *(CONTINUED)*

AREA TO COVER	SPECIFIC QUESTIONS
Nose	Do you have a history of the following? • nosebleeds • nasal obstruction • frequent sneezing episodes • nasal drainage—color, frequency, and amount • trauma or fracture to the nose or sinuses • sinus infection (include treatment received) • allergies • postnasal drip • pain over sinuses • change in the sense of smell • difficulty breathing through nose
Mouth and throat	Do you have a history of the following? • oral herpes infections • mouth pain • difficulty chewing or swallowing • lesions in mouth or on tongue • tonsillectomy • altered taste • sore throat (include dates and frequency) • bleeding gums • toothache • hoarseness or change in voice • dysphagia When did you last have a dental examination? What were the results? What is your daily dental care regiment? Do you wear dentures or any other type of dental appliance?

PHYSIOLOGICAL ASSESSMENT: GENERAL (CONTINUED)

AREA TO COVER	SPECIFIC QUESTIONS
Respiratory system	Do you have a history of any of the following? • asthma • bronchitis • tuberculosis • shortness of breath-if so, preceded by how much and what type of activity • coughing up blood • noisy breathing • pollution or toxin exposure • emphysema • pneumonia • chronic cough • chest pain with breathing • wheezing • smoking How much sputum do you cough up per day? What color is it?
Cardiovascular system	Have you experienced any of the following? • chest pain • heart murmur • need to be upright to breathe, especially at night • swelling in arms or legs • hair loss on legs • anemia • cramping pain in the legs and feet • leg ulcers • palpitations • color changes in fingers or toes • coronary artery disease • varicose veins • thrombophlebitis • coldness, numbness, or tingling in the fingers or toes Do you have hypertension, high cholesterol levels, or a family history of heart failure? Do you smoke? How many packs per day?

PHYSIOLOGICAL ASSESSMENT: GENERAL *(CONTINUED)*

AREA TO COVER	SPECIFIC QUESTIONS
Cardiovascular system *(continued)*	Do you sit or stand for long periods? Do you cross your knees when sitting? Do you use support hose?
Urinary tract	Do you have a history of any of the following? • painful urination • difficulty or hesitancy in starting urine flow • urgency • flank pain • cloudy urine • incontinence • frequent urination at night • pain in suprapubic region • changes in urine • decreased or excessive urine output • kidney stones • blood in the urine • pain in groin • bladder, kidney, or urinary tract infections • low back pain • prostate gland infection or enlargement
Gastrointestinal system	Have you experienced any of the following? • appetite changes • dysphagia • indigestion or pain associated with eating (obtain symptoms) • vomiting blood • ulcers • gallbladder disease • colitis • constipation • black stools • hemorrhoids • food intolerance • heartburn

PHYSIOLOGICAL ASSESSMENT: GENERAL *(CONTINUED)*

AREA TO COVER	SPECIFIC QUESTIONS
Gastrointestinal system *(continued)*	• burning sensation in stomach or esophagus • other abdominal pain • chronic or acute nausea and vomiting • abdominal swelling • liver disease • appendicitis • flatulence • diarrhea • rectal bleeding • fistula How often do you have a bowel movement? Have there been any changes in the characteristics of your stool? Do you use any digestive aids or laxatives? What kind and how often? **THE ELDERLY:** For patients over age 50, obtain the date and results of last Hemoccult test.
Male reproductive system	Do you have a history of any of the following? • penile or testicular pain • penile discharge • hernia • sexually transmitted disease • sores or lesions • penile lumps • prostate gland problems • infertility How often do you perform testicular self-examination? Are you satisfied with your sexual performance? Do you practice safe sex?

PHYSIOLOGICAL ASSESSMENT: GENERAL *(CONTINUED)*

AREA TO COVER	SPECIFIC QUESTIONS
Female reproductive system	Do you have a history of any of the following? • excessive menstrual bleeding • painful intercourse • vaginal itching • bleeding between periods • missed periods • infertility • painful menstruation Provide the following information: • menstrual history, including age of onset, duration, amount of flow, any menopausal signs or symptoms, age at onset of menopause, any postmenopausal bleeding • satisfaction with sexual performance • date of last period • understanding of sexually transmitted disease prevention, including AIDS • number of pregnancies, miscarriages, abortions, stillbirths • date and results of last Pap test • contraceptive practices • vaginal discharge and characteristics

THE ELDERLY:
Ask elderly patients if they have experienced vaginal dryness or other problems.

PHYSIOLOGICAL ASSESSMENT: GENERAL *(CONTINUED)*

AREA TO COVER	SPECIFIC QUESTIONS
Breasts	Have you experienced any of the following? • nipple changes • nipple discharge—color, frequency, odor, amount • rash • breast pain, tenderness, or swelling Have you ever breast-fed? When was your last breast examination? What were the results? Do you perform breast self-examination? When did you last have a mammogram? What were the results? (for women over age 40)
Neurologic system	Do you have a history of any of the following? • seizure disorder, stroke, fainting, or blackouts • weakness, tic, tremor, or paralysis • numbness or tingling • memory disorder, recent or past • speech or language dysfunction • nervousness • mood change • mental health dysfunction • disorientation • hallucinations • depression Do any of these problems affect your day-to-day activities?
Musculoskeletal system	Do you have a history of any of the following? • arthritis or gout • joint or spine deformity • noise accompanying joint motion • fractures • joint pain, stiffness, redness, or swelling (include location, any migration, time of day, and duration)

PHYSIOLOGICAL ASSESSMENT: GENERAL *(CONTINUED)*

AREA TO COVER	SPECIFIC QUESTIONS
Musculoskeletal system *(continued)*	• other pain (include location and any migration) • problems with gait • limitations in motion • muscle pain, cramps, or weakness • chronic back pain or disk disease • problems running, walking, or participating in sports Do any of these problems affect your day-to-day activities?
Immune system	Do you have a history of any of the following? • anemia • low platelet count • blood transfusions (include any reactions) • chronic sinusitis • conjunctivitis • unexplained swollen glands • bleeding tendencies, particularly of skin or mucous membranes • HIV exposure • excessive bruising • fatigue • allergies, hives, itching • frequent sneezing • exposure to radiation or toxic agents • frequent, unexplained infections Do any of these problems affect your day-to-day activities?

PHYSIOLOGICAL ASSESSMENT: GENERAL *(CONTINUED)*

AREA TO COVER	SPECIFIC QUESTIONS
Endocrine system	Do you have a history of any of the following? • excessive urine output • unexplained weakness • changes in hair distribution • hormone therapy • nervousness • inability to tolerate heat or cold • endocrine disease, for example, thyroid or adrenal gland problems, diabetes • increased food intake • excessive thirst • goiter • excessive sweating • tremors • unexplained changes in height or weight • changes in skin pigmentation or texture (In addition discuss the relationship between the patient's weight and appetite.)

PHYSIOLOGICAL ASSESSMENT: CURRENT COMPLAINT

The following table provides a guide to collecting data about the patient's current complaint. Always begin by having the patient describe, in his or her own words, the reason for today's visit.

AREA TO COVER	SPECIFIC QUESTIONS
Time frame	When did the discomfort or alteration in pain start? Is it intermittent or constant? Is it worse at certain times of day?
Location	Where is the pain located? (Have the patient show you.)
Quality	Describe the pain. Is it sharp or dull? How severe is it?

PHYSIOLOGICAL ASSESSMENT: CURRENT COMPLAINT *(CONTINUED)*

AREA TO COVER	SPECIFIC QUESTIONS
Environment	Are there specific places or activities that seem to trigger the pain? Does anything relieve the pain? Make it worse?
Perception	What do you think your symptoms mean?

ASSESSING FUNCTIONAL STATUS

In addition to collecting specific physiological data, you need to assess the patient's ability to function on a day-to-day basis. The table below provides guidelines for such an assessment.

AREA TO COVER	SPECIFIC QUESTIONS
Daily activities	• What do you do during an average day? Does your complaint interfere with this? If so, in what way? • Do you exercise? If so, what type of exercise do you perform and how often do you exercise? Does your complaint interfere with exercise? If so, in what way? • Do you use street drugs? If so, how often? How has this affected you in terms of work and family?
Sleep and rest	• How long do you sleep? Need to sleep? • Do you have any difficulty falling asleep or staying asleep? • Do you wake during the night to urinate? How often? • Do you feel rested each morning? • Do you feel tired during the day?

ASSESSING FUNCTIONAL STATUS (CONTINUED)

AREA TO COVER	SPECIFIC QUESTIONS
Nutrition	• What have you had to eat or drink in the past 24 hours? Is this a typical daily diet? • Who buys and prepares food in your family? • Is the family income sufficient for the family food budget? • Does the family eat together? • How much caffeine from coffee, tea, or soda do you drink in a day? • When did you last have an alcoholic beverage? What do you drink and how much? Have you ever had a drinking problem?
Stress factors	• Do you live alone? • Do you know your neighbors? • Is the neighborhood safe or high in crime events? • Can you keep the temperature in the house comfortably warm or cool? • Are safety factors at work or in the home a stress factor? • What stressors would you list as present in your life now and in the past year? • Has anything about this stress level changed? • Have you ever tried anything to relieve stress? How well did it work?

FAMILY AND SOCIAL ASSESSMENT

It's particularly important to explore the patient's family history and relationships. The health history provides important clues about the patient's state of health and about how family relationships affect treatment and care.

FAMILY ENVIRONMENT

The following table provides questions you can ask the patient that will help build a picture of his or her family environment. However, these questions imply a nuclear family structure. If the patient comes from a single-parent, gay, or extended family, you will need to modify them accordingly.

AREA TO COVER	SPECIFIC QUESTIONS
Mortality data on blood relatives	What is the age and health of your living blood relatives (parents, grandparents, siblings)? At what age did other relatives die and what was the cause of death?
Family history	Is there any family history of diabetes, heart disease, high blood pressure, stroke, blood disorders, cancer, sickle cell anemia, arthritis, allergies, obesity, alcoholism, mental illness, seizure disorder, kidney disease, tuberculosis?
Spouse and children	What are the ages and health condition of your spouse and children?
Patient's position within the family (The purpose of these questions is to find out how tasks are divided within families with children and to explore family health promotion, factorsthat are very important to patient care.)	• Are you happy with the set of tasks that you and your partner do as spouses and as parents? • Are there differences of opinion about child-rearing? How do you work out any differences? • Do you work outside the home? How does the family support you in your work? • Who is the primary caretaker of the children or older adults in the family? Are you happy with this arrangement? • Who makes doctor appointments, keeps track of medication schedules, and so on?

FAMILY ENVIRONMENT (CONTINUED)

AREA TO COVER	SPECIFIC QUESTIONS
Patient's position within the family (continued)	• Are you comfortable with how your children are maturing? Are they learning skills like hygiene, good eating habits, appropriate sleep and rest patterns? • Can family members share or switch tasks? Do they have the skills to do so? • Do you and your children have the same values? • If you are the caretaker, how will your family adjust to your illness?
Patient's views of the economics of the family	• Is your family income adequate to supply its basic needs? • Who makes the money decisions in your family?
Patient's support (These questions will help you understand your patient's social skills, the extent to which the patient has access to a support system, and if the patient is likely to feel isolated and depressed.)	• Do you belong to any clubs or organizations outside the family? What do you enjoy about them? • Whom do you ask for help and advice outside your immediate family? • How do you interact with your co-workers? • What do you like to do with your friends? How often do you get to do it? • Are you happy with your friendships? • What do you know about community agencies that can help you while you are ill and recovering?

FAMILY ENVIRONMENT *(CONTINUED)*

AREA TO COVER	SPECIFIC QUESTIONS
Patient's perception of family	• What is the place of family in your life? • Does your extended family include close friends? • Does anyone who is not a member of your immediate family live in your home? • How do family members interact? • Do they see each other in a positive light? • How do family members react to each other's needs and wants? Are positive and negative feelings expressed openly? • How does the family handle conflicts?

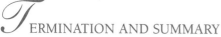

TERMINATION AND SUMMARY

End your interaction with the patient with the following:
- Summarize important information collected during the interview as well as the results of the interview and any conclusions you have drawn from it.
- If there are issues about health education—for example, contraception—either schedule a health education session or provide the patient with the information.
- Make any necessary referrals. Help the patient set up the appointment.
- Summarize decisions you and the patient have made about future care.
- Explain the physical part of the health assessment in detail.
- Ask the patient if he or she has any other concerns or questions.

DOCUMENTING THE INTERVIEW

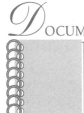

How you document what you have learned from the patient is as important as how you conduct the interview. Other health care professionals will use the patient's record as a basis for future care and treatment. It is important that you allow yourself adequate time to reflect on what the patient has told you and the most effective way to communicate that to other professionals in writing. Observe the following guidelines:

- Use the correct form.
- Use an ink pen, not a pencil.
- Write the patient's name and identification number on each page.
- Make sure the date and time appear with each entry.
- Use standard abbreviations that everyone will understand.
- Wherever possible, use the patient's description of symptoms.
- Wherever possible, be specific, not vague. Do not generalize.
- Do not leave anything blank. If something is not applicable, write "N/A" in that space.
- Do not backdate an entry.
- Never write on a previous entry.
- Never document for anyone but yourself.

Chapter 2. Physical Assessment Skills

▽ ▽ ▽ ▽ ▽ ▽ ▽

INTRODUCTION

SEE TEXT PAGES

In the first chapter we explored techniques for the subjective portion of the health history. In this chapter we explore techniques for the objective portion—the physical assessment. This portion of the assessment will either confirm or bring into question the conclusions you and the patient drew during the subjective assessment. It can generate new avenues of exploration.

TOOLS OF THE TRADE

You yourself provide the most important equipment used in the assessment—your eyes, ears, nose, and fingers. What you see, hear, smell, and touch is critical. You will supplement those tools with special equipment. At a minimum, you will require a measuring tape, penlight or flashlight, thermometer, and visual acuity chart. You will also need additional basic equipment to complete the assessment. (See chart below.)

ASSESSMENT TOOLS

TOOL	USE
Wooden tongue depressor	Assess the patient's gag reflex and obtain a view of the pharynx.
Safety pins	Test the patient's sensation of dull and sharp pain.
Cotton balls	Test the patient's sensation of fine touch.
Test tubes of hot and cold water	Test the patient's ability to distinguish temperature.
Common substances, like coffee or vinegar	Test the patient's ability to smell and taste.

ASSESSMENT TOOLS (*CONTINUED*)

TOOL	USE
Disposable latex gloves	When handling body fluids (taking blood, rectal, and vaginal assessment)
Water-soluble lubricant	Assess rectum and vagina.

SPECIALIZED ASSESSMENT TOOLS

You may find that you need more specialized equipment to complete your assessment. Such equipment may include one or all of the following: reflex hammer, skin calipers, vaginal speculum, goniometer, transilluminator, ophthalmoscope, nasoscope, otoscope, and tuning fork. These tools require additional training to use correctly.

TOOL	DESCRIPTION	USES
Ophthalmoscope	Light source with a system of lenses and mirrors	Examine the internal eye structure: • Use the large aperture for most patients. • If the patient has small pupils, use the small aperture. • Use the target aperture to localize and measure fundal lesions. • Use the slit beam to measure lesion elevation and the anterior eye. • Use the green filter to determine specific fundal details.

!

NURSE ALERT:
You can adjust the intensity of light, but it's best to begin at the lowest level to avoid causing discomfort to the patient.

SPECIALIZED ASSESSMENT TOOLS (*CONTINUED*)

TOOL	DESCRIPTION	USES
Otoscope	Light source similar to the ophthalmo-scope.	Examine the external auditory canal and tympanic membrane.
Nasoscope	Three types: •Nasal speculum •A speculum for the nostrils that you attach to an ophthalmoscope •Handle like an ophthalmoscope, with short, slim head with light source	Examine the nasal interior. **!** **NURSE ALERT:** If you are not skilled in the use of the nasoscope, do not use it. You can cause the patient discom-fort.
Tuning fork	Shaped like a fork. Tines are designed to vibrate.	Check hearing and sensation.

DRAPING AND POSITIONING TECHNIQUES

Before you begin the actual assessment, you need to understand how to position and drape the patient. The correct technique varies, depending on the body area you are assessing. This table provides a quick description of draping and positioning tech-niques.

BODY AREA	POSITION	DRAPING
Head, neck, and thorax	Patient sits on edge of examination table.	None
Neurologic	In some cases, patient needs to to stand or sit.	None

DRAPING AND POSITIONING TECHNIQUES (CONTINUED)

BODY AREA	POSITION	DRAPING
Musculoskeletal	In some cases, patient needs to stand or sit.	None
Breast exam	Phase one: Seated Phase two: Supine, with pillow or towel under the shoulder on the side you are examining; have patient place arm on that side above her head.	None
Abdomen	Supine	Towel over female patient's breasts; for both sexes, sheet draped over lower half of body; do not pull the sheet below the pubic area
Cardiovascular	Supine	Sheet draped over torso and legs
	Sitting	Sheet draped over areas not being auscultated
Rectal (male)	Bent over the examination table or lying on left side	None
Rectal or reproductive (female)	Lithotomy position	Sheet draped over chest and knees and between legs

ASSESSMENT TECHNIQUES

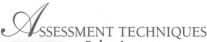

Palpation

You will use palpation, or different kinds of touch, throughout the assessment. Generally, palpation will follow inspection.

It is particularly important to palpate the abdominal or urinary tract systems at the end of the assessment. Otherwise, you may cause the patient unnecessary discomfort and distort findings.

During the assessment, you are likely to use four types of palpation. Light palpation requires a gentle touch with just the fingertips. Do not indent the skin more than 3/4 in (2 cm). If you push too hard, you will dull the sensation in your fingertips.

Deep palpation is more aggressive and usually involves both hands. Depress the skin 1.5 in (4 cm). Place the opposite hand on top of the palpating hand, using it as a control and guide. Use this technique to locate and examine organs such as the kidney and spleen or to anchor an organ like the uterus with one hand while examining it with the other. A variation on this technique involves using one hand to depress the skin and then removing it quickly. If the patient complains of increased pain as you release pressure, you have discovered an area of rebound tenderness.

NURSE ALERT:

If you use this variation during an examination of the abdomen and the patient feels rebound tenderness, consider the possibility that the patient may have peritonitis.

Light ballottement is a variation on light palpation. Using your fingertips, move from area to area, depressing the skin lightly, but quickly. Be sure to maintain contact with the patient so that you can identify tissue rebound.

Deep ballottement is a variation on deep palpation. Using your fingertips, move from area to area, depressing the skin deeply, but quickly. Be sure to maintain contact with the patient's skin.

Percussion

With percussion, you use your fingertips or hands to tap areas of the patient's body. Tapping can be used to make sounds, to find tender areas, or to judge your patient's reflexes. When used for sound, percussion requires specialized training and the ability to distinguish between slight differences in the sounds produced. Move from areas that make clear sounds to dull areas.

There are three percussion techniques: indirect, direct, and blunt.

- Indirect percussion involves both hands. Place the second finger of your left hand if right-handed or your right hand if left-handed against the appropriate body area—for example, the abdomen. Use the middle finger of your other hand to sharply and quickly tap your finger over the body area just below your first joint. Remember to keep the wrist of the tapping hand loose and relaxed.
- Direct percussion uses the hand or fingertip to directly tap a body area. This method is used to find tender spots and to examine a child's thorax.
- Blunt percussion uses the fist, either directly on the body area or on the back of your opposite hand, which is placed on the body area. You use this method to find tender spots. A second type of blunt percussion involves the use of the reflex hammer to create muscle contraction.

NORMAL AND ABNORMAL PERCUSSION SOUNDS

BODY AREA	SOUND	DESCRIPTION
Healthy lung	Resonance	Long, low, moderate to loud, hollow
Hyperinflated lung	Hyperresonance	Long duration, extremely loud and low-pitched, booming

NORMAL AND ABNORMAL PERCUSSION SOUNDS (CONTINUED)

BODY AREA	SOUND	DESCRIPTION
Pleural fluid accumulation or thickening (abnormal)	Dullness	Soft to moderately loud, thud
Abdomen	Tympany	Moderate duration, high-pitched, loud drum-like over hollow organs: stomach, intestine, bladder
	Dullness	Moderate duration, high-pitched, soft to moderately loud, thud
		THE PREGNANT PATIENT: Liver, full bladder, uterus of pregnant woman
Muscle (normal)	Flatness	Short duration, soft, high-pitched, flat

ASSESSMENT TECHNIQUES

Auscultation is the process of listening to the sounds different body areas produce—for example, the heart and lungs. You can hear many body sounds, such as the wheeze of the asthma sufferer, with your ear. Other sounds, such as a heart murmur, require the use of a stethoscope. With the exception of the abdomen, auscultation is the last procedure you conduct in the assessment. When assessing the abdomen, first visually inspect it and then listen for sounds. End the assessment with percussion and palpation. Otherwise, bowel sounds may be disrupted by the examination.

When using a stethoscope, observe the following procedure:
- Conduct the exam in a quiet environment.
- Use a quality instrument with bell and diaphragm with ear pieces that fit you comfortably.
- Expose the body area to which you are listening—fabric can obscure sound.
- Remind the patient not to talk during the procedure, and ask the patient to stay as still as possible.
- Warm the stethoscope head with your hand. If it is cold, the patient may jump or shiver, which will result in extraneous sounds.
- Place the stethoscope head over the body area.
- Close your eyes to eliminate any distractions.
- Listen carefully and develop a complete description of any sound you hear, including how often each occurs.

PERFORMING THE ASSESSMENT

In most cases, you will not have the luxury of conducting the entire assessment. In such cases, gear the assessment to the diagnosis. Use the guidelines in Chapter 1, "Health History," when conducting the assessment.

COMPONENTS OF THE ASSESSMENT

A full assessment is based on the patient's health history (see Chapter 1, "Health History"). You end it with an examination of all the body areas. Note any factors, including race, gender, and age, that may affect a diagnosis. Pay attention to any signs of personal distress. Signs of distress include the following:
- shortness of breath—suggesting a respiratory or cardiac problem
- wheezing or difficulty sitting still—suggesting asthma
- labored breathing—suggesting pneumonia or heart failure
- withdrawn posture, arms crossed, rapid speech, sudden hand movements—suggesting emotional distress
- limited movement, grimacing, clutching the affected area—suggesting pain

NURSE ALERT:
For severe pain, especially in the chest or abdomen, you may need to contact a physician immediately.

Assessing Elderly Patients

When assessing elderly patients, it is more important to explore current complaints than collect a past history. You may also need to modify the assessment if your patient appears confused. In that case, ask simple, direct questions and enlist the aid of someone close to the patient. Otherwise, follow the guidelines in this chapter.

Aging may reduce the body's resistance to illness, tolerance of stress, and ability to recuperate from an injury. It can also cause weakening and stiffening of the muscles; loss of hearing, sight, or the ability to smell; slowing of reflexes; and changes in vital signs.

In some cases, aging may mean a loss of intellectual and reasoning skills. Heart disease, diabetes, cataracts, and cancer are more prevalent among older patients.

It's also important to bear in mind that the elderly patient may be on many different medications. You should always watch such a patient for adverse drug reactions and interactions.

When you assess elderly patients, follow these guidelines:
- Always be respectful of the patient. Establish whether or not the patient is comfortable with conversing on a first-name basis.
- Be sure the patient can understand and follow your explanations and instructions. If not, speak slowly and simply.
- Be patient—the elderly patient may take longer to answer your questions or respond to your suggestions.
- Make sure the patient doesn't have a hearing problem. On the other hand, don't automatically raise your voice.
- Some elderly patients may have to move slowly and will have trouble getting from one position to another during the assessment. Allow them extra time.
- Watch for evidence that the patient is beginning to have difficulty taking care of himself or herself.
- Watch for evidence that the patient is not eating properly.
- Learn to identify the symptoms of age-specific diseases, such as osteoporosis and Parkinson's disease.
- Observe the patient for signs of depression. If an ordinarily neat patient begins to show up for appointments in disarray, depression may be the underlying fac-

tor. Depression can also cause mood swings, irritability, and difficulty paying attention.

- If you observe confusion in the patient, do not assume that it results from changes in the brain. Drugs, poor eating habits, dehydration, and even a change in surrounding and routines can all cause confusion in elderly people.
- Maintain a positive attitude toward normal changes of aging.

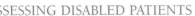

ASSESSING DISABLED PATIENTS

When assessing disabled patients, make any necessary adjustments. For example, a mute patient should be given a written questionnaire. Or, you may need a sign interpreter for a deaf patient. Use simple, direct sentences and questions with an intellectually impaired patient. In any case, it is helpful to have a close friend or relative attend the visit with the patient.

When assessing such a patient, observe the following:
- Adapt your interaction with the patient to his or her abilities.
- Establish to what extent the patient can be a participant in the assessment before you begin. A severely mentally disabled patient may not be able to participate at all. Other patients may require special assistance.
- Be sensitive to the patient's needs and emotional state.
- Pay attention to the patient's feelings about the disability and about the assessment itself.
- Ascertain the patient's level of independence.

TRANSCULTURAL CONSIDERATIONS

Do not confuse cultural differences with abnormal behavior. Before drawing any conclusions, try to get a feel for cultural differences.

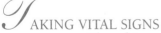

TAKING VITAL SIGNS

The taking of vital signs is fundamental to the physical assessment. Specifically, you check the patient's pulse, respiration, temperature, and blood pressure. Vital signs allow you to establish baseline values for the patient and record changes in the patient's health status. It is preferable to take the signs at once because variations from the norm can indicate possible problems with the patient's health.

A single measure of a vital sign is less reliable than multiple measurements. Ask patients what is normal for them.

If a patient shows an abnormal pattern in a vital sign, make sure that you don't show any apprehension or concern. You should explore any change in vital signs.

NURSE ALERT:
If you take a reading that you think is inaccurate, repeat it. If it still seems inaccurate, have another nurse perform the reading. If you still question the reading, try using a different instrument to check its validity. Explain why you are repeating the measurement.

MEASURING HEIGHT AND WEIGHT

Keeping track of your patient's height and weight is as important as assessing his or her vital signs. When measurements are taken regularly, they help you track the patient's growth and development. If, for example, the patient exhibits a sudden weight loss, this alerts you to the possible onset of illness.

You will also use height and weight in calculating doses of drugs. They are also a way of measuring the success of drugs, fluid, or nutrients administered I.V.

MEASURING PULSE

To take the pulse, you generally use the wrist. If the patient's wrist is injured, or if the patient has diabetes or vascular insufficiency, you will also check all the peripheral pulses to make sure that circulation is normal.

When taking the pulse, palpate the artery for 60 seconds while applying gentle compression. It's less accurate to count for 15 seconds and multiply by 4 because you are likely to miss any abnormalities in heart rate or rhythm.

NURSE ALERT:
If you must use the carotid artery, be extremely careful with the amount of pressure you place on the artery. Too much pressure can trigger reflex bradycardia. Never press on both carotid arteries at once because you can disrupt circulation to the brain.

When taking an infant's or a toddler's pulse, you can either auscultate the apical pulse or palpate the carotid, femoral, atrial, or brachial pulse. You can also take the pulse by watching the movement of the anterior fontanelle.

MEASURING BLOOD PRESSURE

When taking blood pressure, observe the following:

- Check that the patient has not exercised or eaten in the past 30 minutes.
- Make sure that the patient is relaxed.
- Check that the cuff is the right size for the patient. If the cuff is too small, the blood pressure will be falsely elevated; if the cuff is too large, the blood pressure will be falsely lowered.
- Make sure that the bladder is centered over the brachial artery.
- Keep the patient's arm level with the heart by supporting it.
- Listen for pulse sounds as you slowly open the air valve:
  - The beginning of a clear, soft tapping that increases to a thud or loud tap. This is the systolic presssure sound.
  - The change of the tapping to a soft, swishing sound
  - The return of the clear tapping sound
  - A muffled, blowing sound. This is the first diastolic sound. If your patient is a child or physically active adult, this reading is the most accurate reading of diastolic pressure.
  - The disappearance of the muffled, blowing sound. This is the second diastolic sound.

It is more accurate to record the blood pressure readings at the systolic pressure, the first diastolic and the second diastolic sound—for example—110/72/70, although this is not usually done in daily practice.

ASSESSING RESPIRATORY PATTERNS

When assessing respiration, be sure to ascertain the rate, rhythm, and depth.

RESPIRATORY PATTERNS

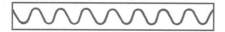

Eupnea
Normal respiratory rate and rhythm

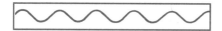

Tachypnea
Increased respiratory rate

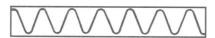

Bradypnea
Slow but regular respirations

Apnea
Periodic absence of breathing

Hyperventilation
Deeper respirations, but at normal rate

ASSESSING REPIRATORY PATTERNS (*CONTINUED*)

RESPIRATORY PATTERNS

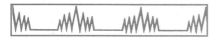

CHEYNE-STOKES
Gradually quickening and deepening respirations, alternating with slower respirations and periods of apnea

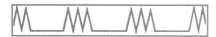

BIOT'S
Faster and deeper than normal respirations of equal depth punctuated with abrupt pauses

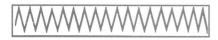

KUSSMAUL'S
Faster and deeper than normal respirations without pauses

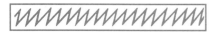

APNEUSTIC
Respirations with prolonged, gasping inspirations followed by very short, inefficient expiration

*C*hapter 3. Head-to-Toe Physical Assessment

▽   ▽   ▽   ▽   ▽   ▽   ▽

*I*NTRODUCTION

SEE TEXT PAGES

This chapter contains a collection of charts that will serve as a guide to assessing the patient from head to toe.

ASSESSMENT TECHNIQUES: HEAD AND NECK

ASSESSMENT	NORMAL FINDINGS	DEVIATIONS FROM NORMAL
Inspect hair, scalp color, and condition.	Normal color; normal texture; full distribution over scalp; scalp pink, smooth, mobile, and free of lesions **THE ELDERLY:** May have thin hair.	Thinning or thickening of the hair—endocrine disorders or side effects from medications; dandruff; dull, coarse, brittle hair; nits
Palpate from the forehead to the posterior triangle of the neck for posterior cervical lymph nodes.	Symmetrical, rounded normocephalic head, positioned at midline, with no lumps or ridges	Note unusual asymmetry, changes in head size, enlarged or painful lymph glands
Palpate around the ears, under the chin, and in the anterior triangle for anterior cervical lymph nodes.	Nonpalpable lymph nodes or small, soft, round, mobile lymph nodes without tenderness	Note the location, size, consistency, tenderness, temperature, and mobility of any enlarged nodes

ASSESSMENT TECHNIQUES: HEAD AND NECK (CONTINUED)

ASSESSMENT	NORMAL FINDINGS	DEVIATIONS FROM NORMAL
Auscultate the carotid arteries.	No bruit on auscultation	Bruit—area of turbulent blood flow
Palpate the trachea.	Straight, midline	Deviation from the midline
Use only one finger to palpate the suprasternal notch.	Palpable pulsations with even rhythm	Abnormal aortic arch pulsations
Palpate the supraclavicular area.	Nonpalpable lymph nodes	Enlarged lymph nodes
Gently palpate the left and then the right carotid artery using the index and middle fingers.	Equal pulse amplitude and rhythm	Unequal pulse amplitude and rhythm

!

NURSE ALERT:
Do not palpate both sides of the anterior neck at the same time. If you accidentally press on both carotid arteries, you may interrupt blood flow to the brain.

ASSESSMENT TECHNIQUES: HEAD AND NECK (CONTINUED)

ASSESSMENT	NORMAL FINDINGS	DEVIATIONS FROM NORMAL
Use the pads of your fingers to palpate the thyroid gland; inside the sternocleidomastoid muscle and below the cricoid and thyroid cartilage.	Thin, mobile thyroid isthmus; non-palpable thyroid lobes	Enlarged or tender thyroid, nodules **!** **NURSE ALERT:** If you find an enlarged thyroid, auscultate for bruits.
Have patient shrug the shoulders against resistance applied by your hands.	Normal range of motion, equal range and strength **THE ELDERLY** May have difficulty tilting the head. Only move the head to the point of discomfort.	Loss of full range of motion
Have patient touch chin to the chest and to each shoulder, touch ear to each shoulder, and tilt head back	Equal strength and movement	Asymmetrical strength or movement
Have patient push left cheek and then right cheek against your hand.	Equal strength and movement	Asymmetrical strength or movement

ASSESSMENT TECHNIQUES: HEAD AND NECK (CONTINUED)

ASSESSMENT	NORMAL FINDINGS	DEVIATIONS FROM NORMAL
Inspect patient's face.	Symmetrical facial features	Edema, lesions, or deformities
Have patient smile, wrinkle forehead, puff cheeks.	Symmetrical in all actions	Asymmetrical in any action
Inspect nose.	Symmetrical and non-deviated; tissue pink and nontender	Edema, deformity, nasal discharge, discoloration, flared nostrils, redness, swelling

NURSE ALERT:
Note color of any mucus.

Alternate holding one nostril shut while patient breathes through the other.	Equal functioning, both passages clear	Inability to breathe through either or both nostrils
Support the patient's head with your free hand and use an ophthalmoscope handle with a nasal attachment to inspect internal nostrils.	Pink mucosa	Inflamed, swollen mucosa; polyps

THE PREGNANT PATIENT:
Nasal mucosa may be mildly swollen.

NURSE ALERT:
Don't use an ophthalmoscope handle with a nasal attachment on an infant or young child. It is too sharp. Use a flashlight for illumination instead.

ASSESSMENT TECHNIQUES: HEAD AND NECK (*CONTINUED*)

ASSESSMENT	NORMAL FINDINGS	DEVIATIONS FROM NORMAL
Gently palpate the nose.	Symmetrical, smooth	Edema, bumps, tenderness, asymmetry
Percuss and palpate the sinuses.	No tenderness	Tenderness. If tender, transilluminate the sinuses.

!

NURSE ALERT:
Prior to age 8, the frontal sinus is too small to percuss or palpate.

Have patient open and close mouth while you palpate temporomandibular joints with your middle three fingers.	Smooth, quiet movement; bones aligned	Misalignment, tenderness, clicking

ASSESSMENT TECHNIQUES: HEAD AND NECK *(CONTINUED)*

ASSESSMENT	NORMAL FINDINGS	DEVIATIONS FROM NORMAL
Inspect interior structure of mouth with tongue depressor and penlight.	Pink mucosa and gingiva	Inflammation, edema

NURSE ALERT:
Have the patient remove any dental prosthetics. Wear gloves.

THE PREGNANT PATIENT
In the pregnant patient, you may find the gingiva to be swollen.

TRANSCULTURAL CONSIDERTIONS:
The mucosa of dark-skinned patients is bluish. This pigmentation is normal.

THE CHILD
A child may have as many as 20 baby teeth. The emergence of baby teeth begins at approximately 6 months. Baby teeth are replaced by secondary teeth between the ages of 6 and 12.

ASSESSMENT TECHNIQUES: HEAD AND NECK (CONTINUED)

ASSESSMENT	NORMAL FINDINGS	DEVIATIONS FROM NORMAL
Inspect the tongue and palates. **NURSE ALERT:** Use this to check hydration in children.	Pink, moist; without ulcers or lesions	Inflammation; lesions; dry, cracked tongue; coated tongue; red inflamed tongue; gingiva on palate
Have patient stick out tongue.	Midline	Cannot hold tongue straight
Have patient stick out tongue and say "Ahh."	Soft palate and uvula rise symmetrically; pink, midline uvula; both tonsils behind pillars	Asymmetry of structures; swollen, inflamed tonsils
Lightly touch back of tongue to test gag reflex. **NURSE ALERT:** If your patient is nauseated, you may want to skip this assessment.	Patient gags; if swallowing is intact, usually gag reflex is present	No gag reflex **NURSE ALERT:** Perform when problem suspected with cranial nerves 9 and 10.

ASSESSMENT TECHNIQUES: HEAD AND NECK *(CONTINUED)*

ASSESSMENT	NORMAL FINDINGS	DEVIATIONS FROM NORMAL
Have patient push against tongue depressor with each side of tongue.	Symmetrical movement and strength	Asymmetry, loss of taste

!

NURSE ALERT:
If patient reports loss of taste, test with cotton swabs dipped in vinegar, sugar, etc. |
| Use a test tube containing a familiar substance, like coffee, to test smell.

!

NURSE ALERT:
Have patient close eyes. | Correctly identifies substance | Unable to identify common substance |
| Test visual acuity using Snellen eye chart.

THE CHILD:
A young child's vision may be 20/30. | 20/20 vision; patients over age 40 may have reduced near vision. | Hesitancy, squinting, vision poorer than 20/30—suggest patient visit an ophthalmologist |

ASSESSMENT TECHNIQUES: HEAD AND NECK *(CONTINUED)*

ASSESSMENT	NORMAL FINDINGS	DEVIATIONS FROM NORMAL
Have patient read newsprint aloud held at a distance of 12 to 14 in (30.5 to 35.5 cm)	Normal near vision	Abnormal near vision—suggest patient visit an ophthalmologist

NURSE ALERT:
Make sure patient wears any corrective lenses.

NURSE ALERT:
If patient is illiterate, use Snellen E chart.

Have patient identify pattern of colored dots on a special color plate.	Identifies pattern; accurate color perception	Cannot identify pattern

NURSE ALERT:
It's very important to diagnose color blindness in a child as early as possible. This gives the child ample time to learn to compensate and alerts parents and other caretakers.

ASSESSMENT TECHNIQUES: HEAD AND NECK (CONTINUED)

ASSESSMENT	NORMAL FINDINGS	DEVIATIONS FROM NORMAL
Perform six cardinal positions of gaze test.	Bilaterally equal eye movement; no nystagmus	Nystagmus **NURSE ALERT:** Refer any patient who cannot pass this test to an ophthamlologist.
Perform cover/uncover test.	Eyes steady; no jerking or wandering eye movement	Wandering, jerking **NURSE ALERT:** Refer any patient who cannot pass this test to an ophthalmologist.
Perform corneal light reflex test.	Eyes steadily fixed on an object Bilateral corneal light reflection	Eyes not parallel when fixed on an object **NURSE ALERT:** Refer any patient who cannot pass this test to an ophthalmologist.

ASSESSMENT TECHNIQUES: HEAD AND NECK *(CONTINUED)*

ASSESSMENT	NORMAL FINDINGS	DEVIATIONS FROM NORMAL
Test peripheral vision.	Normal vision laterally, above, down, and medially, **THE ELDERLY** Patient may have decreased peripheral vision.	Vision deviates from 50 degrees from top, 60 degrees medially, 70 degrees downward, 110 degrees laterally; detects only large defects in peripheral vision
Inspect external eye structures.	Clear, symmetrical eyes; even eyelashes **THE ELDERLY** May have few eyelashes, dull eyes. 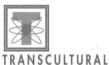 **TRANSCULTURAL CONSIDERATIONS** Asian patients may have eyelids with epicanthal folds.	Cloudy eyes with nystagmus, asymmetry, lid lag, bulging, edema, redness, outward or inward-turning lids, styes, edema, scaling, lesions, unequally distributed eyelashes, eyelashes curve inward, reddened lacrimal apparatus

ASSESSMENT TECHNIQUES: HEAD AND NECK (CONTINUED)

ASSESSMENT	NORMAL FINDINGS	DEVIATIONS FROM NORMAL
Palpate lacrimal apparatus to check tear ducts.	Nontender, pink; without drainage or lumps	Tenderness, masses, too much tearing, drainage

NURSE ALERT:
Culture any drainage.

Examine conjuncti-va and sclera.	Pink conjunctiva with no drainage; clear sclera	Edema, drainage, hyperemic blood vessels, inflammation, conjunctivitis, color changes in sclera, scleral icterus

NURSE ALERT:
Wash hands between examining each eye.

THE ELDERLY
May have pinguecu-la.

TRANSCULTURAL CONSIDERATIONS
Small spots on sclera are normal in dark-skinned patients.

ASSESSMENT TECHNIQUES: HEAD AND NECK *(CONTINUED)*

ASSESSMENT	NORMAL FINDINGS	DEVIATIONS FROM NORMAL
Shine penlight across eye to examine cornea, iris, and anterior chamber.	Clear, transparent **THE ELDERLY** Cornea may have thin, graying ring. **TRANSCULTURAL CONSIDERATIONS** A gray-blue cornea is normal in dark-skinned patients.	Clouding of cornea, portion of iris does not illuminate
Check pupils.	PERRLA: pupils equal, round, reactive to light and accommodation **THE ELDERLY** After age 85 pupils may not react to accommodation.	Asymmetry in size, asymmetrical reaction to light or its absence, fixed pupils, dilated or constricted pupils
Use ophthalmoscope to check red reflex.	Clearly defined orange-red glow	Absence of red reflex—indicative of opacity and clouding

ASSESSMENT TECHNIQUES: HEAD AND NECK (CONTINUED)

ASSESSMENT	NORMAL FINDINGS	DEVIATIONS FROM NORMAL
Check ears.	Line up with eyes, same color as face, symmetrical and proportional to face	Asymmetry, lesions, redness, hard-packed ear wax, drainage, nodules

THE ELDERLY
Reduced adipose tissue and hardened cartilage

TRANSCULTURAL CONSIDERATIONS
Ear wax is yellow in light-skinned patients and dark orange or brown in dark-skinned patients.

Palpate ear and mastoid process.	Absence of pain, tenderness, and swelling	Tenderness, pain, edema, lesions, nodules

NURSE ALERT:
If otitis externa, tenderness, or edema is present, be careful with the otoscope—you may be unable to use it.

ASSESSMENT TECHNIQUES: HEAD AND NECK (CONTINUED)

ASSESSMENT	NORMAL FINDINGS	DEVIATIONS FROM NORMAL
Check hearing in each ear by whispering or holding a ticking watch to the ear.	Normal hearing (whisper from 1 to 2 ft; tick from 5 in)	Loss of hearing

NURSE ALERT:
Note the distance at which you perform the test.

ASSESSMENT	NORMAL FINDINGS	DEVIATIONS FROM NORMAL
Weber's test with tuning fork.	Vibrations heard equally in both ears	Sound heard best in ear with conductive hearing loss
Rinne test with tuning fork.	Equal period of hearing in front of ear and on mastoid process	Conductive or sensorineural hearing loss; vibrations heard longer on mastoid process or front of ear

ASSESSMENT TECHNIQUES: POSTERIOR THORAX

ASSESSMENT	NORMAL FINDINGS	DEVIATIONS FROM NORMAL
Examine the back.	Normal skin tone, symmetry of structure, shoulder height, and inhalation	Asymmetry, accessory muscle use, scoliosis

ASSESSMENT TECHNIQUES: POSTERIOR THORAX (CONTINUED)

ASSESSMENT	NORMAL FINDINGS	DEVIATIONS FROM NORMAL
Examine the antero-posterior and lateral thorax.	2:1 relationship between lateral and anteroposterior diameter	Increased diameter indicative of pulmonary disease
THE CHILD Measure chest circumference at nipples.	**THE ELDERLY** Diameter ratio may normally increase.	
Palpate the spine.	Straight alignment Firm, symmetrical	Abnormal alignment, lesions, tenderness, asymmetrical muscles, pain
Palpate the posterior thorax.	Normal, smooth	Lesions, lumps, pain, inflammation, abnormalities
Percuss the costovertebral area.	Normal thud	Pain, tenderness

ASSESSMENT TECHNIQUES: POSTERIOR THORAX *(CONTINUED)*

ASSESSMENT	NORMAL FINDINGS	DEVIATIONS FROM NORMAL
Inspect respiratory function.	Symmetrical expansion and contraction	Asymmetry
Palpate as patient says "99" over and over.	Symmetrical vibration Note: Vibration varies over chest.	Increased vibration
Percuss systematically over the lung area.	Resonant over lungs and dull over diaphragm	Asymmetrical sounds, dull over lungs, hyperresonance (pulmonary disease)

THE CHILD
An infant's chest is too small for reliable percussion.

THE ELDERLY
Hyperresonant sounds possible from hyperinflation of lung tissue.

ASSESSMENT TECHNIQUES: POSTERIOR THORAX (CONTINUED)

ASSESSMENT	NORMAL FINDINGS	DEVIATIONS FROM NORMAL
Percuss each side of posterior thorax for diaphragmatic excursion.	1¹/₄ to 2¹/₄ in excursion **NURSE ALERT:** The right side of the diaphragm is usually higher than the left.	Unequal excursion
Have patient take slow, deep breaths through mouth while you systematically auscultate the lungs. **THE CHILD** Auscultate a child first—other procedures may cause crying. **NURSE ALERT:** If the patient has a great deal of chest hair, moisten it to reduce interference.	Bronchial, vesicular, and bronchovesicular sounds **THE CHILD** A child may normally have coarser lung sounds.	Wheezing, coarse to fine crackles, rhonchi **NURSE ALERT:** Crackles may indicate congestive heart failure.

ASSESSMENT TECHNIQUES: ANTERIOR THORAX

ASSESSMENT	NORMAL FINDINGS	DEVIATIONS FROM NORMAL
Inspect anterior thoracic area.	Normal skin tone, symmetry of structures and inhalation	Abnormal skin tone, accessory muscle use, asymmetry, deformity, lifts, heaves, or thrusts, point of maximum impulse visible
	!	**!**
	NURSE ALERT: Children and men breathe with their diaphragm muscles, adult women breathe with their upper chest.	**NURSE ALERT:** Children and very thin patients may normally have visible point of maximum impulse.
Palpate anterior thorax.	No tenderness or lesions	Lesions, lumps, pain, left and right symmetry
Inspect respiratory excursion.	Symmetrical expansion and contraction	Asymmetrical expansion and contraction

ASSESSMENT TECHNIQUES: ANTERIOR THORAX (*CONTINUED*)

ASSESSMENT	NORMAL FINDINGS	DEVIATIONS FROM NORMAL
Palpate as patient repeats "99" over and over. **THE CHILD** Unreliable in an infant.	Resonant lung fields, dullness over bony structures **THE ELDERLY** May have hyperresonant sounds.	Dullness over lung fields, abnormal sounds over bony structures
Perform a breast exam. **NURSE ALERT:** Have a patient with large, pendulous breasts lean forward.	Soft, symmetrical breasts, symmetrical nipples **THE PREGNANT PATIENT** Breasts are swollen, nipples dark, areola dark, may have purple streaks.	Asymmetry, abnormal hair growth, lesions, lumps, nodes, thickening; cracks, fissures, blisters, inflammation, pain, etc. **NURSE ALERT:** Culture any nipple discharge.
With patient at 45 degree angle, inspect jugular veins.	No pulsation	Distended, changes in bounding pulse

ASSESSMENT TECHNIQUES: ANTERIOR THORAX *(CONTINUED)*

ASSESSMENT	NORMAL FINDINGS	DEVIATIONS FROM NORMAL
Palpate precordium.	Point of maximum impulse at apical area	Shift in point of maximum impulse indicates abnormal changes in left ventricle
Auscultate for heart sounds.	S_1 and S_2, normal rhythm, pulse rate normal for age	Extra heart sounds, murmurs, rubs **THE CHILD** A child may have benign heart murmurs.

ASSESSMENT TECHNIQUES: ABDOMEN

ASSESSMENT	NORMAL FINDINGS	DEVIATIONS FROM NORMAL
Inspect abdomen.	Normal contour for body type and age, normal skin color	Asymmetry, bulges, visible growths, abnormal color, rash, visible peristaltic waves, hernia, lesions

ASSESSMENT TECHNIQUES: ABDOMEN (*CONTINUED*)

ASSESSMENT	NORMAL FINDINGS	DEVIATIONS FROM NORMAL
Systematically auscultate abdomen for up to 5 minutes in all four quadrants	Normal bowel sounds in all areas	Bruits, other abnormal sounds; hyperactive sounds in one area followed by absent sound

NURSE ALERT:
Auscultate before percussion or palpation. If you perform either procedure first, you may generate abnormal sounds or rupture an aneurysm.

Percuss on left and right side from just below breast to midclavicular line.	Dull over liver, tympanic over abdomen	Abnormal sounds

NURSE ALERT:
You may not feel the liver border if the patient has gas in the colon or congestion in the right lower lung.

ASSESSMENT TECHNIQUES: ABDOMEN (*CONTINUED*)

ASSESSMENT	NORMAL FINDINGS	DEVIATIONS FROM NORMAL
Systematically palpate abdomen, moving from upper to lower areas in each quadrant. **NURSE ALERT:** It helps a ticklish patient to place a hand over yours while you palpate.	Soft, nontender symmetrical abdomen	Tenderness, masses, pain, bladder distention **NURSE ALERT:** Examine any painful area last to prevent the patient from tensing to guard the area.
Palpate the liver.	Often nonpalpable; if edge palpable, smooth, nontender	Mushy, enlarged, lumps
Palpate the spleen.	Nonpalpable	Palpable (enlarged)
Palpate femoral groin pulse. **THE CHILD** This is an important pulse point in children.	Symmetrical, strong	Asymmetrical, weak or absent **NURSE ALERT:** Absent pulse with blue extremities is a clinical emergency.

ASSESSMENT TECHNIQUES: UPPER EXTREMITIES

ASSESSMENT	NORMAL FINDINGS	DEVIATIONS FROM NORMAL
Inspect the upper extremities.	Normal, uniform skin color and texture, symmetrical muscle mass, good skin turgor	Abnormal color or texture, lesions, dryness, asymmetrical muscle mass, poor skin turgor

THE CHILD
Skin turgor on the upper extremities and chest is important for identifying dehydration in infants and young children.

THE ELDERLY
Skin may be dry and thin with deficient turgor.

Have patient turn palms up and down with arms extended.	Steady hands, symmetrical movement	Tremors, pronator drift, unable to follow instructions
Have patient push forearms up and down against your hand.	Symmetrical strength and movement	Asymmetry when comparing left to right
Inspect and palpate all joints.	Normal range of motion	Stiffness, edema, enlarged joint, redness, pain with movement, limited range of motion

ASSESSMENT TECHNIQUES: UPPER EXTREMITIES *(CONTINUED)*

ASSESSMENT	NORMAL FINDINGS	DEVIATIONS FROM NORMAL
Palpate hands for temperature.	Warm, moist, symmetrical	Cool, clammy skin or warm, dry skin; asymmetry
Palpate brachial pulses.	Right and left equal	Decreased pulse strength, thready pulse, difference between right and left pulse
Inspect fingernails.	Color, shape, and condition normal, good capillary refill	Broken and cracked nails, pitting, clubbing, cyanosis, decreased capillary refill
Have patient squeeze two of your fingers with each fist.	Symmetry in hand strength	Asymmetry

ASSESSMENT TECHNIQUES: LOWER EXTREMITIES

ASSESSMENT	NORMAL FINDINGS	DEVIATIONS FROM NORMAL
Inspect lower extremities.	Even skin color and texture, symmetrical muscle mass, hair and nail growth	Abnormal color, lesions, dryness, hair loss, bruises, varicosity, edema, fungal toe nails, asymmetrical muscle mass

ASSESSMENT TECHNIQUES: LOWER EXTREMITIES (*CONTINUED*)

ASSESSMENT	NORMAL FINDINGS	DEVIATIONS FROM NORMAL
Palpate for pitting edema between knee and ankle and in foot.	No edema	Pitting edema present— grade according to scale
Palpate posterior tibial area and dorsalis pedis.	Symmetrical pulse, skin temperature	Asymmetrical, weak, or absent pulse; skin temperature decreases **!** NURSE ALERT: If any pulse is abnormal, check the popliteal pulse.
Perform the straight leg test on each leg.	Normal movement THE ELDERLY May have difficulty with this test.	Pain with extension **!** NURSE ALERT: Help a patient with difficulty extending by steadying leg.

ASSESSMENT TECHNIQUES: LOWER EXTREMITIES *(CONTINUED)*

ASSESSMENT	NORMAL FINDINGS	DEVIATIONS FROM NORMAL
Palpate hip with abduction and adduction.	No crepitus	Crepitus

THE CHILD
Use Ortolani's maneuver on an infant.

ASSESSMENT	NORMAL FINDINGS	DEVIATIONS FROM NORMAL
Have patient raise each thigh against your hand; push tibial area out against your hand; pull calf back against your hand.	Symmetrical strength	Weak or asymmetrical strength

THE CHILD
Test strength by having child hop on each leg.

𝒮UGGESTED READINGS

Anderson, F. D., and J. Malone. "Taking Blood Pressure." *Nursing94* 24 (November 1994): 34–39.

Flory, C. "Perfecting the Art of Skin Assessment." *RN* 55 (June 1992): 22–27.

Hartrick, G., and A. E. Lindsey. "Family Nursing Assessment: Meeting the Challenge of Health Promotion." *Journal of Advanced Nursing* 20 (July 1994): 85–91.

Jensen, L., and M. Allen. "Wellness—The Dialectic of Illness." *Image, Journal of Nursing Scholarship* 2 (Fall 1993): 220–224.

Chapter 4: Anatomy and Physiology Review

▽   ▽   ▽   ▽   ▽   ▽   ▽

INTRODUCTION

SEE TEXT PAGES

The nervous system is a highly complicated network of nerves governed by the brain and directed through the vertebral column. This chapter provides an overview of the anatomy and physiology of the nervous system.

ANATOMY AND PHYSIOLOGY

The three basic components of the nervous system are the central nervous system (CNS; the brain and spinal cord, the operating centers of the system), peripheral nervous system (nerves that extend throughout the body from the spinal cord to receive and transmit information; includes cranial nerves and spinal nerves), and autonomic nervous system (regulator of bodily functions that occur automatically or without any conscious thought).

These systems are further divided into smaller subsystems, each with a specific function that can be affected by disease or trauma.

Specialized Cells: The Building Blocks of the Nervous System

The primary cells in the nervous system are neurons, which send and receive information. The four types of neurons are motor, sensory, internuncial, and cortical. All neurons have the same basic structure, including a cell body (place in which chemical reactions occur that direct a cell's functions), dendrites (projections from the cell body that receive impulses and transmit this information to the cell body), and an axon (a long projection that carries impulses away from the cell body either directly to an organ, to another neuron, or to the dendrites of another neuron).

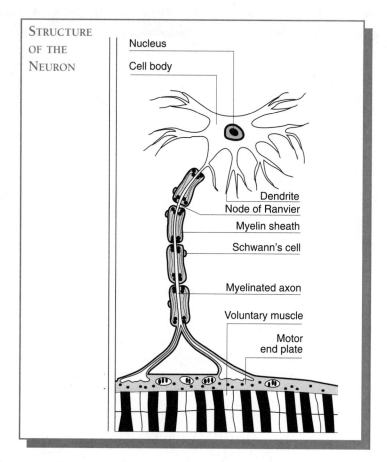

Structure of the Neuron

Nucleus

Cell body

Dendrite
Node of Ranvier
Myelin sheath
Schwann's cell
Myelinated axon
Voluntary muscle
Motor end plate

Neurons in the CNS are protected by myelin, a fatty, white substance that helps to improve the transmission of impulses. Neurons outside the CNS have an additional covering, a sheath of Schwann's cells, also called the neurilemma. The neurilemma, a key component of cell regeneration, helps myelin to form and also stimulates the axon to regenerate if it is cut. Neurons in the CNS cannot regenerate independently because they are not surrounded by neurilemma.

Transmission of Impulses

A neuron transmits impulses by responding to a stimulus that changes the electrical charges within a cell. This stimulus is provided by neurotransmitters, chemical substances that alter the chemical balance of the cell to transmit information across synapses (spaces between the axon and the next neuron over which the nerve impulse passes) and send the impulse through the neuron. Acetylcholine is the main neurotransmitter; other neurotransmitters include dopamine, serotonin, norepinephrine, and gamma-aminobutyric acid. After transmission of a nerve impulse, the cell returns to its original chemical balance so that another impulse can be transmitted; this interval is known as the refractory period.

The neuroglia are the nervous system's supporting tissue cells. Types of neuroglia include astrocytes (provide structure, help regulate chemicals that surround neurons, provide nourishment to neurons), oligodendrocytes (form the myelin sheath), microglial cells (responsible for phagocytosis), and ependyma (assist in manufacturing cerebrospinal fluid (CSF), protect cerebral tissue from infiltration by foreign substances). Unlike neurons, neuroglial cells can reproduce through mitosis (rapid division of one cell into two or more). Neuroglial cells outnumber neurons by a rate of 10 to 1. CNS tumors often are made up of neuroglial cells and can be considered a form of neuroglial overgrowth.

The Brain

The main divisions of the brain are the cerebrum, cerebellum, limbic system, and brain stem. Other significant structures include the basal ganglia, thalamus, hypothalamus, and pituitary gland (see Other Structures of the Brain, page 74).

The cerebrum, the largest section of the brain, is divided down the center by a longitudinal fissure into the right and left hemispheres; these hemispheres communicate through the corpus callosum, a band of white connecting fiber that joins them at the base of the fissure. Each hemisphere controls functions on the opposite side of the body, a process called contralateral control. Gyri are folds created on the surface of the hemispheres that increase the brain's surface area; the folds are separated by fissures called sulci. Each hemisphere is divided into four lobes that govern aspects of physical, emotional, and cognitive functioning; the lobes can include more areas with specific responsibilities (see Lobes and Their Functions).

Anatomy of the Brain

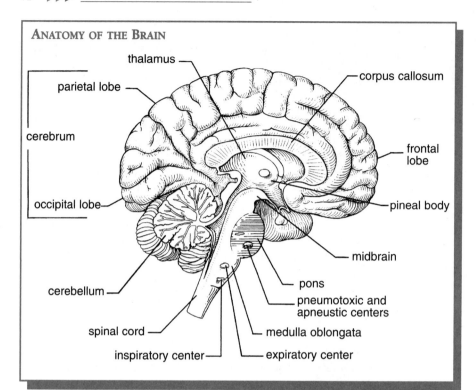

Lobes and Their Functions

Frontal lobe

- Prefrontal area: controls such autonomic activities as breathing, GI processes, circulation, and pupillary movements; in conjunction with limbic system, governs personality and helps regulate higher processes, such as thought, concentration, and logical abilities
- Prerolandic-precentral gyrus: governs voluntary motor movement
- Broca's motor speech area: controls speech; typically located in the dominant hemisphere
- Written speech area: usually in the left hemisphere; governs the ability to write
- Primary motor area: responsible for individual movements of different parts of the body

Temporal lobe
- Controls memory and identifies the qualities of sound; place where long-term auditory associations are stored
- Wernicke's second motor speech area: works with the temporal lobe to aid in interpretation of spoken and written language

Parietal lobe
- Postcentral gyrus: governs sensory areas and processes information from the spinal cord
- Speech area: based on individual's dominant hemisphere; recognizes pain, temperature, pressure, and positions of body and limbs; governs ability to sense by touch

Occipital lobe
- Controls vision and stores long-term visual associations

The cerebellum controls functions necessary for movement, such as posture and balance, speed and acceleration, fine motor activities, and the ability to execute repetitive and sequential movements. The cerebellum is divided into two hemispheres similar to those of the cerebrum, except that each hemisphere controls body function on its respective side (known as ipsilateral control).

The limbic system is the operating center for emotions and basic survival drives; it consists of the anterior nucleus of the thalamus, amygdaloid nucleus, hypothalamus, hippocampal formation, cingulate gyrus, mamillary bodies, and subcallosal area.

The brain stem, located next to the cerebellum further inside the cranium, is divided into three sections: midbrain, pons, and medulla oblongata. Ten of the 12 cranial nerves also originate in these three sections. (See Cranial Nerves, page 80.)

The midbrain, the topmost portion of the brain stem, is a relay point for impulses from nerve centers above and below it. It includes the tubular aqueduct of Sylvius, which carries CSF between the third and fourth ventricles of the brain.

The pons, the central part of the brain stem, governs normal respiration through the pneumotaxic center and shares responsibility with the medulla oblongata for the excitatory cardiovascular center.

The medulla oblongata, the third section of the brain stem that sits just above the spinal cord and below the pons, controls the inhibitory cardiovascular center and the inspiratory respiratory center, which govern such reflexes as gagging, swallowing, and coughing.

The reticular activating system (RAS), which works with the thalamus and hypothalamus to maintain alertness, also functions from the medulla oblongata. The RAS integrates nerve impulses from throughout the CNS and transmits them to different parts of the CNS as indicated and is also responsible for sleep and wakefulness patterns and other biological cycles.

The brain requires 20% of the blood circulating through the body. Four main arteries feed the brain: two vertebral and two carotid. The vertebral arteries, rising from the subclavian arteries, join together at the front of the brain to create the basilar artery. The basilar artery, in turn, divides into the posterior cerebral arteries. The internal carotid arteries rise from the common carotid arteries, which, in turn, rise from the aortic arch.

All of the major arteries are connected at the base of the brain by the circle of Willis, an anastomosis that ensures continuation of blood circulation if any arteries become blocked. Blood circulates back into the body through openings in the dura mater called sinuses. These sinuses grow increasingly larger and eventually empty into the jugular vein.

OTHER STRUCTURES OF THE BRAIN

This chart features some important structures in the brain, including those that protect and nourish the brain (skull, meninges, ventricular system, blood-brain barrier).

STRUCTURE	DEFINITION/ LOCATION	FUNCTION
Basal ganglia	Also known as extrapyramidal system; consists of several parts	Controls initiation of movement

OTHER STRUCTURES OF THE BRAIN *(CONTINUED)*

STRUCTURE	DEFINITION/ LOCATION	FUNCTION
Thalamus	Center of cranium behind frontal lobes of cerebrum	Directs impulses from peripheral nerves of body to appropriate points in rest of brain; involved in sensory awareness of pain
Hypothalamus	Just under thalamus	Regulates body temperature and certain metabolic processes, such as appetite, by secreting hormones and controlling the autonomic nervous system; plays a role in control of emotions; works in conjunction with pituitary gland to regulate water metabolism
Pituitary gland	Small endocrine gland connected to hypothalamus by pituitary or hypophyseal stalk; divided into anterior (adenohypophysis) and posterior (neurohypophysis) lobes	Controls other endocrine system glands; influences metabolism and physical development by secreting hormones

The brain, which is nourished by the cerebrovascular system, is encased and protected by the cranium, which is made up of the skull, meninges, ventricular system, and blood-brain barrier.

OTHER STRUCTURES OF THE BRAIN *(CONTINUED)*

STRUCTURE	DEFINITION/ LOCATION	FUNCTION
Skull	Consists of bones of cranium and face: 14 facial bones; 8 cranial bones (2 parietal, 2 temporal, frontal, occipital, sphenoid, ethmoid); names correlate to portion of brain they protect; bones are connected by immovable joints called sutures (four main sutures [sagittal, coronal, basilar, lambdoid])	Protect the brain
Meninges	Contains three layers: dura mater (outer, thickest layer; separated from skull by epidural space), arachnoid (middle layer; separated from dura mater by narrow subdural space), and pia mater (thin; adheres tightly to brain and spinal cord; separated from arachnoid layer by subarachnoid space, location of brain's larger blood vessels); also houses foramina, openings through which brain's nerves and blood vessels pass	Three layers cover and protect the brain, spinal cord, and blood vessels that serve the brain; foramina permit circulation of CSF between brain and spinal cord

OTHER STRUCTURES OF THE BRAIN (CONTINUED)

STRUCTURE	DEFINITION/ LOCATION	FUNCTION
Ventricular system	Consists of four ventricles	Manufactures and distributes CSF, which provides a cushioning layer, acts as lymphatic system for brain and spinal cord, and creates a stable environment for cells in CNS; CSF, constituted primarily of protein, salt ions, and sugar, is manufactured in clusters of capillaries, called choroid plexuses (located in brain's ventricles), that manufacture between 500 and 700 mL of CSF a day; about 150 mL circulates through system at one time
Blood-brain barrier	Capillary membrane; less well developed in children, making them generally more susceptible to organisms in bloodstream than are adults	Prevents toxic substances from moving out of capillaries and into extracellular fluid; increased intracranial pressure diminishes effectiveness of blood-brain barrier and increases likelihood of cerebral cells being threatened by toxic substances

Spinal Cord and Vertebral Column

The spinal cord, the chief messenger for the body, transmits nerve impulses to the brain from the extremities and organs of the body and sends nerve impulses back to the body's periphery from the brain. The spinal cord also acts as a reflex center; therefore, assessment of damage to particular areas of the nervous system can be based on whether certain reflexes remain intact after injury or illness. Contained within the vertebral column, the spinal cord has a specific structure that allows nerve impulses to pass through it.

Vertebrae, the bones of the vertebral column, protect the spinal cord and provide the skeletal structure to enable body structure and movement. The vertebral column has five sections, with a set number of vertebrae in each: cervical, 8 pairs; thoracic, 12; lumbar, 5; sacral, 5; and coccygeal, 1. The number of spinal nerves corresponds to the number of vertebrae.

The upper two cervical vertebrae (the atlas and the axis) connect to the base of the skull and permit the head to move. The ribs are attached to the body by the 12 thoracic vertebrae; the 5 large lumbar vertebrae support most of the weight of the upper body. Ligaments also connect muscle and skeletal structures to the vertebrae and help to keep the vertebrae aligned. If ligaments are damaged, then the spinal cord and nerves may be as well.

Each vertebrae has a foramen from which the spinal nerves exit and enter. An intervertebral disk made up of cartilaginous tissue pads the bodies of the cervical, thoracic, and lumbar vertebrae. This tissue cushions the vertebrae and spinal cord against shock. The intervertebral disk has two sections: the thick outer annulus and the softer inner nucleus pulposus.

SPINAL CORD AND VERTEBRAL COLUMN ANATOMY

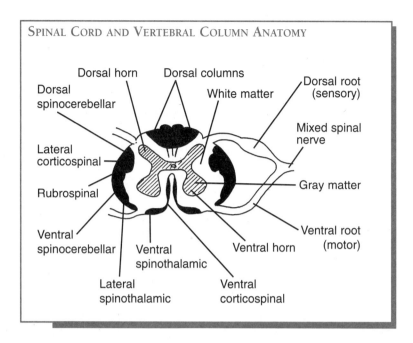

The spinal cord starts at the medulla oblongata and occupies about the first two thirds of the vertebral column. It extends from the 1st cervical vertebra (the atlas) typically to the 12th thoracic or 1st or 2nd lumbar vertebra. The spinal cord is protected by the dura mater, arachnoid, and pia mater and is nourished by the radicular arteries (which enter at the spinal nerve) and the anterior and posterior spinal arteries. Unlike the brain, the spinal cord has no collateral system to protect it in case blood flow is interrupted.

Spinal nerves called the cauda equina (or horse's tail) continue past the actual central canal of nerve tissue and exit from the foramina in the bottom third of the vertebral column (lumbar, sacral, and coccygeal sections). As it reaches past the end of the thoracic vertebrae, the spinal cord narrows into the conus medullaris and then into the filum terminale, a nonneural fiber that attaches to the coccyx.

The nerve tracts in the spinal cord convey sensory (afferent) and motor (efferent) information and direction. The principal sensory tracts convey information as follows: lateral spinothalamic, pain and temperature changes; posterior columns (fasciculus gracilis, fasciculus cuneatus), tactile and body movement; and ventral spinothalamic, touch. The motor tracts convey impulses for voluntary motor movement; the lateral corticospinal (pyramidal) tract (and sometimes the vertical corticospinal tract) acts as the main transmitter for these impulses. The reticulospinal and vestibulospinal tracts (the extrapyramidal system), which originate in the basal ganglia, either encourage or inhibit muscle movement.

Peripheral Nervous System

The peripheral nervous system comprises the nerves (cranial, spinal, large nerve structures throughout the body) that reside in the periphery of the body, away from the CNS. These nerves receive direction from the CNS and send information back.

CRANIAL NERVES

All but the first and second cranial nerves originate in the brain stem. Some have sensory functions and others have motor functions. All cranial nerves work on the same side of the body from which they originate. This chart lists the cranial nerves as well as their number, function, and type.

NUMBER	NAME	FUNCTION	TYPE
I	Olfactory	Smell	Sensory
II	Optic	Vision	Sensory
III	Oculomotor	Upward and medial eye movements (extraocular); pupillary constriction	Motor
IV	Trochlear	Downward eye movement (extraocular)	Motor
V	Trigeminal (ophthalmic, maxillary, mandibular)	Chewing and jaw movements (motor); skin of scalp and face; corneal sensation; mouth and nose mucous membranes (sensory)	Motor and sensory

CRANIAL NERVES (CONTINUED)

NUMBER	NAME	FUNCTION	TYPE
VI	Abducens	Lateral eye movement (motor)	Motor
VII	Facial	Muscles of facial expression and lacrimal and salivary glands (motor); taste in front two thirds of tongue and skin around ear (sensory)	Motor and sensory
VIII	Acoustic	Hearing; sense of balance	Sensory
IX	Glossopharyngeal	Saliva production from parotid glands (motor); taste in back third of tongue; sensations in throat (sensory)	Motor and sensory
X	Vagus	Swallowing; thoracic and cardiac muscles; abdominal organs; secretory glands of pancreas and gastric tract; soft palate; larynx and pharynx (motor); sensation in pharynx, larynx, chest, neck, and abdomen (sensory)	Motor and sensory
XI	Spinal accessory	Pharyngeal and laryngeal movement; shoulder and neck movement; heart muscles (motor); sternocleidomastoid and trapezius area (sensory)	Motor and sensory

CRANIAL NERVES (CONTINUED)

NUMBER	NAME	FUNCTION	TYPE
XII	Hypoglossal	Tongue; muscles for speech (motor); placement of tongue (sensory)	Motor and sensory

Spinal Nerves

The 31 pairs of spinal nerves are named according to the vertebrae by which they exit from the spinal cord and are also numbered according to the vertebral number. The spinal nerves are as follows: cervical nerves (8 pairs; numbered C1 to C8); thoracic nerves (12 pairs; numbered T1 to T12); lumbar nerves (5 pairs; numbered L1 to L5); sacral nerves (5 pairs; numbered S1 to S5); and coccygeal (1 pair).

Autonomic Nervous System

The ANS maintains the body systems that function automatically, or without conscious intervention. It transmits messages to the pupils for dilation and constriction and to certain glands (for example, the thyroid) for hormone secretion to organs (for example, stomach and heart) to maintain, increase, or decrease organ function. The ANS is also responsible for the body's chemical and emotional responses in stress situations. Although systems in the ANS typically function automatically, we have learned how to regulate body functions once thought to be unaffected by conscious processes (for example, blood pressure) by using biofeedback and other mental processes.

The ANS is divided into the sympathetic and the parasympathetic nervous system. The parasympathetic nervous system (PNS) controls basic body functions. The sympathetic nervous system (SNS) governs the body's use of energy and the body's reactions in times of stress or high energy requirement. Parasympathetic fibers originate in the sacral sections of the spinal cord and in cranial nerves III, VII, IX, and X. Sympathetic nerve fibers originate from the cervical and thoracic sections of the cord.

In the SNS, postganglionic nerve fibers release norepinephrine when they reach their destination. This form of adrenaline speeds up body functions. The PNS relies on acetylcholine, the neurotransmitter that slows body processes and conserves energy. The PNS conserves energy and the SNS expends energy in times of stress; therefore, they can have opposite effects on the same organ or gland. Nevertheless, the two work together to create a balance.

EFFECTS OF AUTONOMIC STIMULATION

ORGAN	SNS EFFECT	PNS EFFECT
Pupil	Dilates	Constricts
Salivary gland	Promotes thick secretion	Promotes thin secretion
Heart	Increases rate	Decreases rate
Sweat glands	Produces secretions	Does not produce secretions
Lungs	Constricts blood vessels; dilates bronchi	Constricts bronchi
Penis	Ejaculation	Erection
GI muscle	Inhibits peristalsis, stimulates sphincters	Stimulates peristalsis, inhibits sphincters
Skeletal muscle vessels	Constricts	Dilates

Chapter 5: Subjective Data Collection

▽   ▽   ▽   ▽   ▽   ▽   ▽

Introduction

SEE TEXT PAGES

Your nursing judgment is called into instant action when a patient presents with signs and symptoms of a neurologic problem. Because of the emergency nature of many neurologic conditions, you may need to eliminate history taking and quickly intervene to implement treatment. The degree of your assessment depends on the patient's complaint or presenting problem and on limiting factors such as the patient's level of consciousness (LOC) and physical condition (for example, degree of strength or weakness). You should also be aware of special considerations when gathering information on children and elderly patients.

A complete neurologic assessment covers the following areas: vital signs, mental status, emotional status, LOC, cranial nerve function, motor function, sensory function, and reflexes.

THE CHILD

When collecting data for children, consider the following:

- Consult parents or guardians about any recent changes in the child's behavior and cognitive skills, including school performance and level of play, or changes in sleep-wake patterns. Ask about the child's attention span and any excessive fears.
- Consider the child's judgment and abstract reasoning, which varies with the level of development but becomes more reliable after the child has completed several years of grade school.
- Memory testing is not usually effective until age 4; always use simple words and numbers for young children.
- Attentiveness in infants and young children is best judged by response to the mother, awareness, and parents' responses to any changes. Set up games or play activities to gain further responses from young children.
- Use the Denver Developmental Screening Test on children from birth to age 6 to assess personality and language skills development in the appropriate time frame.

THE ELDERLY

When collecting data for the elderly, consider the following:

- Elderly patients may naturally demonstrate slower thought processes and slower responses to questions meant to show status of cognitive functions, such as memory and judgment. They may also show more general forgetfulness and less need for sleep.
- Elderly patients are more likely than younger patients to become confused because of certain physical conditions, such as dehydration, infection, and hypoglycemia. Sudden confusion, however, usually indicates a neurologic condition. Also, greatly or suddenly deteriorated intellectual capacity or personality patterns can indicate a nervous system disorder.

𝒮UPPORTING ASSESSMENT DATA

The following signs and symptoms may indicate that your patient has a neurologic disorder:

Health History:

- Headache
- Dizziness
- Seizures
- Fainting spells
- Pain
- Numbness and tingling in extremities
- Numbess and tingling in face
- Twitching
- Spasms and tremor
- Muscle weakness (general, specific, one-sided)
- Changes in gait
- Deficits in balance and coordination
- Loss of bowel or bladder functioning
- Changes in sexual functioning (for example, lack of sensation, reduced functioning; with peripheral nerve damage, impotence)
- Nausea and vomiting
- Stiff neck
- Problems chewing and swallowing
- Difficulty talking (for example, using tongue, finding words, writing, using numbers)
- Memory deficits
- Confusion or agitation
- Drooping eyelids
- Ringing in ears
- Changes in vision (for example, blurred or double vision)

- General behavioral changes
- Hallucinations
- Disorientation

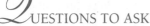

UESTIONS TO ASK

History of Present Illness:

In assessing the patient's present illness, you must first determine the chief complaint, as well as other signs and symptoms and pertinent information. The chief complaint should be in the patient's own words. When taking a history of the patient's present illness, ask the following questions:

- When did the problem begin?
- What are your symptoms?
- How frequently do they occur? Are they becoming more or less frequent?
- Do any events, situations, conditions, or activities precede the onset of symptoms?
- What relieves the symptoms? How long does this relief last?
- Have the symptoms worsened, improved, or stayed the same?
- Have you experienced nausea or vomiting? If so, do you vomit forcefully (projectile) and/or suddenly?

If the patient states that the symptoms have come on suddenly, ask the following questions:

- Have you recently been involved in an accident, hit your head, or fallen? Do you have trouble maintaining your balance?
- Do you sometimes stumble into objects and/or people?
- Have you needed to lean on something for support so you wouldn't fall?
- Have you had any blackouts or felt suddenly dizzy? Did the dizziness occur after changing positions, such as getting out of bed, bending, or picking something up?
- Have you recently fainted? What were you doing when you fainted?

Past Medical History:

When assessing past medical history, including family and social data, ask the following general questions:

- Do you have allergies?
- Have you previously had or do you now have any illnesses, particularly neurologic (such as meningitis), congenital abnormalities, or psychiatric disorders?
- Do you have a history of heart disease, diabetes, hyper-

tension, kidney problems, cancer, asthma, lung disease, anemia, thyroid problems, or GI problems?
- Do you have a history of seizures or headaches?
- Do you smoke or have you ever smoked?
- Do you drink alcohol? What type? How often? How many drinks over how long?
- Do you use recreational drugs? What type? How often? For how long?
- Describe your work or household environment, particularly any stress or possible exposure to chemicals or hazardous waste.
- Do you have a family history of neurologic or psychiatric disorders?

Medication History:

When assessing the patient's medication history, ask the following questions:
- What medications are you currently taking? What medications have you taken in the past 5 years?
- Specifically, are you taking any analgesics, sedatives, hypnotics, antipsychotics, antidepressants, or nervous system stimulants? Have you taken any of these medications in the past 5 years?

QUESTIONS TO ASK: NEUROLOGIC SYMPTOMS

Use these guidelines for questioning your patient about the following neurologic symptoms: headache, sensory or physical changes, seizures, and cognitive and personality changes.

SYMPTOM	QUESTIONS TO ASK
Headache	• Where is the pain? How long does it last? Is it constant or intermittent? • How would you describe the pain: dull, sharp, throbbing? • How intense is the pain on a scale of 1 to 10, with 1 as "little pain" and 10 as "extremely intense pain"? • What time of day does the pain occur? • What activities are you engaged in when the pain occurs? Are you working, at home, active, at rest? • How frequently do the headaches occur? • What do you do to relieve the pain? How long does the relief last? • Do you feel nauseated? Do you need to vomit at these times?

QUESTIONS TO ASK: NEUROLOGIC SYMPTOMS *(CONTINUED)*

SYMPTOM	QUESTIONS TO ASK

Sensory or physical changes

- Have you noticed any changes in your vision, such as blurring, sensitivity to light, double vision, or altered field of vision (for example, not able to see as far to one side as previously)?
- Have you experienced any facial pain, twitching, numbness, weakness, or paralysis (drooping)? Any numbness, tingling, and/or pain in your extremities (hands, feet, arms, and legs)?
- Have you experienced any difficulty eating or swallowing? Any difficulty drinking, resulting in drooling?
- Have you had any spasms or weaknesses in the neck area?
- Have you had any changes in your ability to hear? Any ringing in the ears?
- Have you ever injured yourself without knowing how you did it and without feeling it?
- Have you experienced any changes in your sense of taste or smell?
- Have you experienced any sexual changes or dysfunction?
- Have you experienced any loss of bowel or bladder functioning?

Seizures

- Have you ever had any seizures? At what age did they begin? How many have you had?
- What happens just before the seizures? Do you experience any changes in vision, hearing, and/or smell?
- How long do the seizures last?
- How often do they occur in terms of hours, days, months, or years?
- What is the sequence of events during the seizure? For example, do you see an aura, fall to the ground, cry, have difficulty with motor skills, lose consciousness, or experience incontinence?
- Have you ever taken medication for seizures? If so, what kind and what dosage?

QUESTIONS TO ASK: NEUROLOGIC SYMPTOMS (CONTINUED)

SYMPTOM	QUESTIONS TO ASK
Cognitive and personality changes	• Have you ever had a period of time in which you had speaking difficulty, such as suddenly being unable to speak, inability to find the correct term or name, or speaking gibberish? • Have you experienced any episodes of confusion or memory loss or had the feeling that time had passed but you were unaware of its passage? • Have you experienced mood shifts and/or been unusually irritable? • Have family members or friends commented on changes in your personality? • Have your sleeping patterns changed? • What types of coping mechanisms do you use? (Examples may be significant relationships, counseling, exercise, and support groups.)

THE INTERVIEW

You can also obtain information about a patient's condition by observing how the patient answers your questions and by paying attention to his physical appearance when he answers them. Use this chart as a guide in interviewing your patient.

STATUS	CONSIDERATIONS
Consciousness	• Consider the patient's responses to your questions; patients who are fully conscious respond to questions easily and in a short period of time. • Assess responses and cooperation to routine questions about health concerns and personal history data. • A patient experiencing any change in consciousness may be irritable, confused by your questions, unable to focus for more than short periods of time, unable to orient himself to the environment, or unable to follow basic commands, such as "look up" or "raise your hand."

THE INTERVIEW (CONTINUED)

STATUS	CONSIDERATIONS
Outward appearance	• Observe how patient appears during the assessment. • Consider the following: Is patient appropriately dressed? (Attire should be proper for the weather and suggest personal taste rather than a lack of judgment about what is appropriate.) Groomed properly? (Poor or inappropriate grooming can signal a deficiency or lack of judgment.)
Emotional state	• Observe patient's mood. • Consider the following: What is patient's mood? Is he anxious or irritable? Is patient's mood consistent with what he is saying and with recent occurrences? (For example, a person under great stress may show a flat affect.) Does patient's mood vary for no obvious reason? • Ask patient what makes him angry or sad. (Abnormally hostile, evasive, angry, tearful, or withdrawn replies can indicate a deficit or a psychotic disorder. Also consider if such replies signal potential suicidal or homicidal impulses.)
Cognitive state	A patient with a neurologic deficit may indicate problems with thinking and expression of thoughts and feelings. The inability to communicate is known as aphasia. Aphasia is classified by the type of communication deficit involved. • Receptive aphasia is the inability to understand the spoken and written word. Wernicke's aphasia specifically describes the inability to understand the spoken word, whereas alexia aphasia specifically describes the inability to understand the written word. • Expressive aphasia is the inability to express oneself through speech or writing. Broca's aphasia specifically describes the inability to express oneself through speech, whereas agraphia specifically describes the inability to express oneself through writing. • Global aphasia is a combination of receptive and expressive types of aphasia. The following questions will help you evaluate apha-

THE INTERVIEW (CONTINUED)

STATUS	CONSIDERATIONS
Cognitive state (continued)	sia and other cognitive defects.

• Does patient express complete thoughts? Do the thoughts logically follow one another?
• Can patient follow directions?
• Are patient's perceptions of a situation (for example, the place in which you are talking, the reason for your questions) similar to your own?
• Is patient confused?
• How are patient's speech patterns? Are the rhythms and tone consistent and natural? Does patient increase and decrease volume in a natural and con- sistent manner? Important: Note these responses during longer, more open-ended questions in which patient must formulate a reply.

Ask patient to answer or perform the following to help you more closely assess his cognitive status:
• How is your health? Why are you seeking medical treatment?
• Interpret this saying. (Use familiar sayings, such as "A penny saved is a penny earned." Determine if patient's response is concrete and relevant to the statement. Consider patient's cultural background when selecting a saying.)
• Calculate the following mathematical problems without paper or pencil. (Give patient simple prob- lems, such as adding 8 to 30 and then 9 to that number. Consider patient's level of education.)
• Answer the following association questions. (Ask questions such as "A bark is to a dog as a meow is to a what?" or "Soup is to a bowl as coffee is to a what?" Remember to consider patient's cultural background.)

Memory	To assess patient's memory, ask specific types of ques- tions and compare the answers with normal findings.

• To test recall, ask patient to repeat a series of num- bers in order and then in reverse. Normal recall is five to eight numbers in a series and four to six numbers in reverse.
• To test short-term memory, name three objects and ask patient to repeat what you have said. Patient should be able to repeat the words immediately. Later in the interview ask patient to again repeat

THE INTERVIEW (CONTINUED)

STATUS	CONSIDERATIONS

Memory
(continued)

these words. A normally functioning person should
be able to recall these objects.
- Test recent memory by asking patient to relate
events that have just occurred. For example, ask
patient when he had his last meal and what it was.
Patient should be able to relay this information with
little hesitation. Check the accuracy of the answers
with family members or friends.
- Ask patient long-term memory questions, such as
his telephone number, birthday, the name of the
state you're in, and who the current president is.
Patient should be able to readily offer this information.

Motor function-
ing

- Note the way patient moves and speaks.
- Assess patient's posture. Is it relaxed and natural or
tense, awkward, or slumped?
- Is patient's gait coordinated? Does he stagger or
stumble?
- Are patient's movements smooth, or spastic and
awkward?
- Does patient alter his position in a natural way and
in a normal time period?
- Does patient exhibit any tremor or nervous tics?
- Does patient have any facial drooping or twitches?

Related Diagnoses
The following conditions may affect the neurologic system
or present symptoms similar to those of neurologic disorders:
- depression
- alcohol or drug abuse
- suicide attempts. (If a patient is potentially suicidal, take
precautions to ensure his or her safety.)
- psychotic illness

Chapter 6: Objective Data Collection

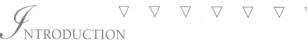

INTRODUCTION

SEE TEXT PAGES

To obtain objective data about your patient, you need to use specific tools, tests, and procedures to collect the information. This chapter is a guide to the physical assessment of the neurologic patient. The list below gives you an overview of the most important signs and symptoms you may find in the neurologic patient. Remember, however, that because of the critical nature of many neurologic conditions (such as acute head injury or cerebrovascular accident [stroke]), you may need to institute emergency treatment measures before performing a full neurologic assessment.

Quick Reference for Objective Assessment Findings
• Abnormal temperature
• Hypertension
• Pulse changes
• Abnormal respirations
• Changes in level of consciousness
• Paresthesia
• Dysphasia
• Aphasia
• Ataxic gait
• Dyskinesia
• Change in muscle reflexes
• Loss of survival reflexes, such as cough, gag, oculocephalic, and oculovestibular
• Tinnitus
• Change in visual fields
• Loss of vision
• Pupillary changes

TOOLS OF THE TRADE

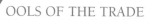

Use the following tools and equipment in the neurologic assessment:
• Watch
• Sphygmomanometer
• Stethoscope
• Penlight
• Tuning fork
• Reflex hammer

- Cotton ball or wisp of cotton
- Cotton-tipped applicator
- Paper clip or safety pin
- Sugar
- Salt
- Test tubes or glasses of both hot and cold water
- Tongue blade
- Ophthalmoscope
- Aromatic substance, such as coffee, peppermint, or lemon
- Reading material
- Snellen's chart
- Pencil
- Pupil gauge
- Otoscope
- Tape measure
- Key
- Paper towel or waxed paper
- Three different-sized coins

ASSESSING NEUROLOGIC FUNCTIONING

Areas you typically may examine include cranial nerves, cerebellar functioning, motor functioning, sensory functioning, reflex responses, and related systems and structures.

ASSESSING THE 12 CRANIAL NERVES

Use the following chart as a guide to assessing the 12 cranial nerves. With children, as appropriate, use games or imitation to draw desired responses.

CRANIAL NERVE/ ASSESSMENT	NORMAL FINDINGS	DEVIATIONS FROM NORMAL
I (OLFACTORY) TOOLS: AROMATIC SUBSTANCES, PENLIGHT		
• Examine each nostril with the penlight to make sure there are no obvious blockages.	Identifies scents correctly	Can't identify odors correctly
• Ask the patient to occlude one nostril and inhale through the other; then have him repeat the process on the other side.		

ASSESSING THE 12 CRANIAL NERVES *(CONTINUED)*

CRANIAL NERVE/ ASSESSMENT	NORMAL FINDINGS	DEVIATIONS FROM NORMAL

I (OLFACTORY) *(CONTINUED)*

- Hold up the aromatic substance. Have the patient occlude one nostril, close eyes, and then identify the odor; repeat with the other nostril. Use more than one aromatic substance, but don't use strong, potentially irritating odors, such as alcohol.

THE ELDERLY
Remember that the ability to see, hear, taste, and smell can naturally decrease with age.

II (OPTIC)
(NOTE: REQUIRES SEVERAL TESTS BECAUSE VISUAL ACUITY, VISUAL FIELDS, AND INTERNAL EYE STRUCTURES ARE ASSESSED.)
TOOLS: NEWSPAPER OR MAGAZINE, SNELLEN'S CHART, PENCIL, PENLIGHT, OPHTHALMOSCOPE

Visual Acuity

- Have patient sit in a well-lighted room, cover one eye, and read Snellen's chart from 20 ft (6 m). Note the smallest line the patient can read (with glasses, if applicable).
- Test both of the patient's eyes, with and without corrective lenses.
- If Snellen's chart is not available, hold up two or three fingers and have patient identify the number.

If vision normal, can read 20/20 line or can identify correct number of fingers

Can't read portions of chart or identify number of fingers

ASSESSING THE 12 CRANIAL NERVES (CONTINUED)

CRANIAL NERVE/ ASSESSMENT	NORMAL FINDINGS	DEVIATIONS FROM NORMAL

II (OPTIC) (CONTINUED)

Visual Acuity (continued)

- Use the newspaper or other reading material to test a patient's near vision. Test each eye individually, as in the Snellen's chart exercise.

THE CHILD
Use Snellen's E chart, a picture chart, or a picture book to assess visual acuity.

Visual Fields

- Stand about 2 ft (0.6 m) away from patient and instruct him to cover one eye. Cover your own opposite eye, so that both of you are looking at the same side of the room.
- Hold an easily recognizable object (for example, a pencil) at arm's length above the patient and then lower it into patient's field of vision.
- Instruct patient to tell you when he first sees the pencil and compare this with the point at which you first see the pencil. You should both see it at the same time. Repeat procedure on opposite eye.

Follows moving object or fingers to edge of visual field with ease

Specific areas of vision are decreased or absent; half of visual field may be blocked out; possible blind spot or contralateral blindness in lower quadrants (inner and outer aspects) of eyes

ASSESSING THE 12 CRANIAL NERVES *(CONTINUED)*

CRANIAL NERVE/ ASSESSMENT	NORMAL FINDINGS	DEVIATIONS FROM NORMAL
Visual Fields *(continued)*		
• Or, have patient face you and look at your nose. Use your hands to test each eye and both eyes together by moving your fingers in from eight different directions into quadrants of patient's vision. If patient appears to have trouble seeing your fingers, move them with a flickering motion and note if patient blinks.		
Internal Eye Structure		
• Seat patient in darkened room. • Using ophthalmoscope, examine fundus (retina and optic disk), blood vessels around optic nerve, and physiologic cup.	Transparent retina; yellow, round or oval optic disk (located where retina and optic nerve converge); blood vessels should surround optic nerve; small, yellow physiologic cup located within optic disk	Enlarged, pink (from blood) optic disk (from papilledema, or choked disk, because optic nerve is swollen); whitish optic disk with no blood vessels surrounding optic nerve; physiologic cup seems too small and patient has vision loss

ASSESSING THE 12 CRANIAL NERVES *(CONTINUED)*

CRANIAL NERVE/ ASSESSMENT	NORMAL FINDINGS	DEVIATIONS FROM NORMAL

III (oculomotor), IV (trochlear), and VI (abducens)
Work together to control eye movement; oculomotor nerve also controls pupil and eyelid movement
Tools: pencil, pupil gauge, penlight

Eyeball Movement

• Look at patient's eyeballs straight on, from the side, and from above the head; compare for any differences in position.	Eyeballs are comparable to one another	One or both eyeballs protrude (proptosis or exophthalmos) or recede abnormally (enophthalmos)

Eyelid Status

• Ask patient to look straight ahead. • Note the width of the space between the upper and lower eyelids from the outer to the inner canthus (the palpebral fissure). • Note eyelid position in relation to pupil and iris.	Eyelids should cover no more than one third of iris	Upper eyelid droops (ptosis); possible edema in upper or lower eyelid from trauma to orbit of eye

Extraocular Movement

• To assess, test for the six cardinal fields of gaze. • Hold your fingers 12 inches (30 cm) in front of patient's nose. • Tell patient to follow movement of your fingers with his eyes only and to keep his head still.	Visualize eye with a cross-hatch over it; eye movement in any direction should bring edge of iris into center of cross-hatch	Involuntary movements, such as oscillation and sudden jerks (nystagmus) or eyes not tracking together

ASSESSING THE 12 CRANIAL NERVES (*CONTINUED*)

CRANIAL NERVE/ ASSESSMENT	NORMAL FINDINGS	DEVIATIONS FROM NORMAL
Extraocular Movement (*continued*)		
• Slowly move your fingers in direction of one of the cardinal fields for about 2 ft (0.6 m). Note point at which patient's gaze stops; repeat for remaining cardinal fields of gaze.		
Extrinsic Eye Movement		
• Stand in front of patient; hold your fingers about 18 inches (45 cm) from patient's nose. Note patient's ability to focus on the fingers. • Next, assess patient's eyes for accommodation and convergence. Tell patient to hold head still, then move your fingers slowly toward patient's nose.	Both eyes converge at same time and pupils constrict; patient can continue staring at your fingers until they're within about 3 inches (7.5 cm) of nose	Eyes converge differently or not at all
Pupil Quality		
• Note size and shape of each pupil and whether they're equal in size. • Use pupil gauge (100-mm ruler) to measure pupils.	Similar size and shape; depending on light in room, pupils will measure in normal range (1.5 to 6 mm)	Unilaterally dilated, fixed, and nonreactive; unilateral, small, and nonreactive; bilateral, dilated, fixed, and nonreactive; bilateral, mid-size, and nonreactive; bilateral, small, and usually nonreactive

ASSESSING THE 12 CRANIAL NERVES *(CONTINUED)*

CRANIAL NERVE/ ASSESSMENT	NORMAL FINDINGS	DEVIATIONS FROM NORMAL
Direct Light Reflex		
• Darken room and have patient cover one eye; hold opposite eye open with your hand. • Direct penlight into pupil at an angle; repeat with other eye.	Pupil constricts immediately and remains that way until light is removed	No immediate constriction or reaction to light
Consensual Light Reflex		
• Darken room; angle penlight to side of one eye; assess reaction of other eye. • Repeat procedure for other eye.	Both pupils constrict bilaterally while light is on	Pupils don't constrict together

V (TRIGEMINAL)

GOVERNS FACIAL SENSATIONS, CORNEAL REFLEX, AND ABILITY TO CHEW; HAS THREE BRANCHES (OPHTHALMIC, MAXILLARY, MANDIBULAR)

TOOLS: WISP OF COTTON, REFLEX HAMMER, TWO TEST TUBES OR SMALL BOTTLES, HOT AND COLD WATER, PAPER CLIP OR SAFETY PIN

Facial Sensations		
• Instruct patient to keep eyes closed. • Touch your fingers to one side of patient's forehead and then the other; ask patient where he feels it. Repeat on both of the patient's cheeks and both sides of jaw simultaneously.	Can identify soft touch of cotton and hot, cold, sharp, and dull sensations	Decreased sensation or absence of sensation on one side

ASSESSING THE 12 CRANIAL NERVES *(CONTINUED)*

CRANIAL NERVE/ ASSESSMENT	NORMAL FINDINGS	DEVIATIONS FROM NORMAL

Facial Sensations *(continued)*

- Next, fill one test tube with cold water and hold it against side of patient's face for about 1 second; ask patient what he feels and where sensation is coming from. Repeat with test tube filled with hot water, then repeat entire sequence on other side of patient's face.
- Next, use sharp end of safety pin or paper clip to touch one side of patient's forehead; touch the same side with the dull end. Repeat with both sharp and dull edges on patient's cheeks and jaw.

NURSE ALERT
Do not test child's superficial pain response with needles; allow child to point to area being touched rather than naming it.

Corneal Reflex

- Instruct patient to look up.
- Hold one eyelid open, touching cornea softly with wisp of cotton; don't touch eyelashes, conjunctiva, or sclera. Repeat on other eye.

Blinking, tearing

No blinking or blinking in only one eye; no tearing

ASSESSING THE 12 CRANIAL NERVES (CONTINUED)

CRANIAL NERVE/ ASSESSMENT	NORMAL FINDINGS	DEVIATIONS FROM NORMAL

Chewing and Jaw Muscles

- Have patient clench teeth while you palpate the temporal muscles (at right and left temples).
- With patient's teeth still clenched, palpate the masseter muscles (on side of jaw joints).
- To test pterygoid muscle strength, ask patient to open his mouth; place one of your hands on patient's head and the other under his jaw. Tell patient to hold jaw open while you try to close it.
- Use reflex hammer to test masseter (jaw jerk) reflex. Tell patient to relax jaw; tap the middle of his chin with the hammer.

Temporal and masseter muscles equal in size and contract bilaterally; during pterygoid muscle test, patient can easily resist pressure to close jaw; slight opening of jaw with jaw jerk test

Muscle groups contract asymmetrically or not at all; irregular facial movements; facial pain; during pterygoid muscle test, patient closes jaw; no response to jaw jerk test, or mouth falls open

THE CHILD
Use food treats to assess jaw function.

ASSESSING THE 12 CRANIAL NERVES (*CONTINUED*)

CRANIAL NERVE/ ASSESSMENT	NORMAL FINDINGS	DEVIATIONS FROM NORMAL

VII (FACIAL)
GOVERNS FACIAL EXPRESSIONS AND SENSE OF TASTE ON ANTERIOR TWO THIRDS OF TONGUE
TOOLS: COTTON-TIPPED APPLICATOR, SUGAR, SALT

Motor Components

• First, observe patient's face during speech and at rest to determine any abnormalities or asymmetry. • Ask patient to raise eyebrows, frown, smile, puff out his cheeks, repeat a one-syllable word, and purse lips and try to whistle. • To test the upper motor component of the face, have patient close eyes tightly. Try to open patient's eyes by gently pulling up the skin above the forehead with your fingers. • To test the lower motor component, have patient puff out his cheeks. Put your fingers on either side of patient's face and try to collapse the cheeks. Tell patient to try to resist your efforts.	Symmetrical facial expressions; patient can execute all expressions; patient resists efforts to open eyes and collapse cheeks	Asymmetrical facial expressions; patient can't execute expressions; patient can't resist external movements of eyes and cheeks

Sensory Function

• Dip cotton-tipped applicator into sugar and ask patient to extend his tongue.
• Touch sugar to each side of anterior part of tongue; tell patient to keep tongue out until he can identify flavor.

ASSESSING THE 12 CRANIAL NERVES *(CONTINUED)*

CRANIAL NERVE/ ASSESSMENT	NORMAL FINDINGS	DEVIATIONS FROM NORMAL
Sensory Function *(continued)*		
(Closing the mouth may move the substance to another part of the tongue.) • Repeat the process with the salt.	Correctly identifies each taste	Cannot identify tastes
VIII (ACOUSTIC) DIVIDED INTO TWO BRANCHES: COCHLEAR (GOVERNS HEARING) AND VESTIBULAR (GOVERNS BALANCE) TOOLS: OTOSCOPE, TUNING FORK, WATCH **Examination for Physical Abnormalities**		
• Examine patient's ear canals for any obvious blockages or physical malformations. Also check for excessive cerumen (earwax), which may interfere with balance or hearing.	No blockages in ear canal; eardrum is pearly or pink disk with malleus handle pointing downward in center of eardrum; in left ear, cone of light in lower right-hand section of left eardrum and lower left-hand section of right eardrum	Bulging, recessed, or inflamed eardrum; ear canal blockage; lack of visualization of light

ASSESSING THE 12 CRANIAL NERVES *(CONTINUED)*

CRANIAL NERVE/ ASSESSMENT	NORMAL FINDINGS	DEVIATIONS FROM NORMAL
Hearing		
• Hold a ticking watch (not quartz or electronic) within 2 inches (5 cm) of patient's ear and ask him to identify the sound; or rub your fingers together by the patient's ears (both ears simultaneously and each separately). • Gradually move watch away from ear and ask patient to identify when sound is no longer audible.	Can hear watch until it's 4 to 6 inches (10 to 15 cm) away	Can't hear or can only slightly hear watch; sound is audible only on one side
Lateralization		
• Use Weber test to detect any hearing deficit on one side. • Vibrate the tuning fork; place it at the center of patient's forehead; ask patient if tone is centralized or louder on right or left side.	Volume and intensity of tone are equal (Weber negative)	Louder tone in right ear (Weber right); louder tone in left ear (Weber left)

THE CHILD
Allow child to point to side that is louder.

ASSESSING THE 12 CRANIAL NERVES (CONTINUED)

CRANIAL NERVE/ ASSESSMENT	NORMAL FINDINGS	DEVIATIONS FROM NORMAL
Sound Conductivity		
• With the Rinne test, you'll use a tuning fork to assess how well the patient hears sound via bone and air conduction. • Vibrate the tuning fork and touch its base to patient's right mastoid process. Note how long it takes patient to no longer hear the tone. • Vibrate the tuning fork again and hold it about 1/2 inch (1.25 cm) from the external ear canal of one ear. (Make sure the prongs are in front of but not touching the canal.) • Ask patient when he hears the sound and then when it's no longer audible.	Immediately hears tone through both bone and air; a tone carried by air conduction is audible much longer than one carried by bone	Cannot hear tone at all or cannot hear tone when fork is held up to ear canal, but can sense vibration at the bone (as long as middle ear is intact)
Equilibrium		
• Examination of vestibular functions is not usually undertaken in the neurologic assessment unless the patient has a history of vertigo, disturbed balance, or tinnitus. Then, oculovestibular testing is used.	Not applicable	Not applicable

ASSESSING THE 12 CRANIAL NERVES *(CONTINUED)*

CRANIAL NERVE/ ASSESSMENT	NORMAL FINDINGS	DEVIATIONS FROM NORMAL
IX (GLOSSOPHARYNGEAL) AND X (VAGUS) MEET AT THE PHARYNX AND GOVERN GAG AND PALATAL REFLEXES; GLOSSOPHARYNGEAL NERVE ALSO CONTROLS TASTE ON POSTERIOR ONE THIRD OF TONGUE TOOLS: TONGUE BLADE, COTTON-TIPPED APPLICATORS, SUGAR, SALT		
Vagus Nerve • Ask patient to yawn or say "ah" to observe the inside of his mouth. • Check soft palate and uvula for upward movement and back of pharynx for inward movement. • Next, ask patient to sit up straight and slowly drink a clear fluid to prevent the patient from aspirating any of the fluid. • Ask patient to say the letters m, b, p, t, and d and the number 1 to evaluate for dysphagia, tongue and palate problems, and difficulty pronouncing statements with alliteration. Evaluate the voice for hoarseness, softness, nasal quality, and clarity.	Both sides of soft palate rise equally; uvula rises; smooth, uninterrupted swallowing movement; speech is of normal tone and clarity	Sides of soft palate don't rise or rise asymmetrically; uvula doesn't rise; awkward, choked swallowing; hoarseness can indicate paralysis of vocal cords; whispery speech can indicate larynx nerve disorder; nasal speech can result from soft palate paralysis; slurring of letters can indicate a motor deficit of the tongue or speech muscles
Gag and Palatal Reflexes • Ask patient to open mouth; hold down patient's tongue with a tongue blade. • Use the cotton-tipped applicator to touch the sides of the pharynx.	Intact gag reflex (occurs immediately when sides of pharynx are touched); uvula rises when touched	Gag reflex not present; uvula remains static

ASSESSING THE 12 CRANIAL NERVES *(CONTINUED)*

CRANIAL NERVE/ ASSESSMENT	NORMAL FINDINGS	DEVIATIONS FROM NORMAL
Gag and Palatal Reflexes *(continued)*		
• Ask patient to open mouth; depress the tongue with the tongue blade, and touch both sides of the uvula with the cotton-tipped applicator.		
Taste Sensation		
• Have patient close eyes, open mouth, and stick out tongue. • Apply a small amount of sugar to the back third of the tongue. Repeat this procedure with salt.	Correctly identifies taste	Cannot identify taste
XI (SPINAL ACCESSORY) INNERVATES TRAPEZIUS AND STERNOCLEIDOMASTOID MUSCLES, WHICH ENABLE HEAD TO ROTATE AND NOD		
• To test trapezius muscle, face patient and place your hands on his shoulders. Ask patient to shrug while you apply downward pressure on the shoulders. • To test sternocleidomastoid muscles, place your hand on one side of patient's face and have him turn against the resistance from your hand. Repeat for other side of head.	Normal strength and ability to resist in these muscles	Overall weakness or differences in one side compared with the other

ASSESSING THE 12 CRANIAL NERVES (*CONTINUED*)

CRANIAL NERVE/ ASSESSMENT	NORMAL FINDINGS	DEVIATIONS FROM NORMAL
XII (HYPOGLOSSAL) GOVERNS TONGUE MOVEMENT TOOL: TONGUE BLADE • Ask patient to open mouth. Observe patient's tongue at rest; then have him stick it out. • Next, ask patient to move tongue as quickly as possible from side to side outside of mouth to assess patient's ability to move tongue (for example, in eating). • To test lingual strength, hold a tongue blade in patient's mouth and have patient press against it with the tongue. Repeat on other side.	Tongue should lie flat at rest; be centered between lips when stuck out; smooth and natural side-to-side movements; has strength and control to move tongue within mouth against pressure	Tongue shows involuntary movement, tremor, or increased wrinkling at rest; falls to one side when stuck out; awkward movements of tongue when outside of mouth; doesn't have strength to press tongue against blade

ASSESSING CEREBELLAR FUNCTIONING

The following tests, which were designed to determine how well the nerves and nerve pathways are conducting information to the extremities, help to assess coordination and balance.

ASSESSMENT TECHNIQUE	NORMAL FINDINGS	DEVIATIONS FROM NORMAL

Hand-eye coordination

• Ask patient to extend right arm and then touch the right index finger to his nose. Then have him return the arm to the extended position and repeat the procedure with the other hand. Finally, have patient repeat entire process with eyes closed.

• Position your finger about 18 inches (0.5 m) in front of patient's nose. Ask patient to extend his right hand to touch your finger and then to touch his nose. Have patient repeat procedure while you reposition your finger several times, then have him repeat entire process with left hand.

Can hold arms extended steadily for 20 seconds; movements are smooth; patient can accurately touch his nose and your finger

THE ELDERLY
Elderly patients may exhibit a slight swaying during tests for standing with eyes closed. They may also have a slow reaction time that could make their movements seem less smooth or rhythmic.

Arm involuntarily moves downward; awkward, uncoordinated movements; cannot touch his nose or your finger; misses his nose

ASSESSING CEREBELLAR FUNCTIONING *(CONTINUED)*

ASSESSMENT TECHNIQUE	NORMAL FINDINGS	DEVIATIONS FROM NORMAL
Hand and arm coordination		
• Have patient sit down, hold hands over thighs with palms down, and quickly and repeatedly pat the thighs. Next, ask patient to turn palms up and alternate quickly patting thighs with palms up and down. • Have patient hold up right hand and touch thumb to each finger in order as quickly as possible; then repeat process with left hand. (Note: Patient may be faster with dominant hand.)	Quick, natural movements; maintains regular rhythm during patting exercise	Jerky, uncoordinated movements; can't pat thighs rhythmically
Foot and leg coordination		
• Have patient lie down and rest left heel on right knee, then slide heel down shin. Repeat process with right heel on left knee. • With patient lying down, stand at end of bed and position your right hand about 4 inches (10 cm) from his left foot. Ask patient to touch your hand with his foot. • Have patient sit on edge of bed and use his right foot to make an imaginary figure eight. Instruct patient to do this for about 30 seconds and then repeat process with left foot.	Has control over movement; smooth, quick, coordinated movements	Cannot move heel smoothly down shin, meet your hand with either foot, or move either foot easily in figure eight pattern; awkward movements

ASSESSING CEREBELLAR FUNCTIONING *(CONTINUED)*

ASSESSMENT TECHNIQUE	NORMAL FINDINGS	DEVIATIONS FROM NORMAL
Balance		
• Have patient stand (without shoes) with feet together and arms at each side; note posture and balance. • Instruct patient to close eyes; again, note posture and balance. • Next, have patient stand on each foot, one at a time and then hop on each foot one at a time.	Can stand with minimal swaying (even with eyes closed), maintain balance for 5 seconds when standing on only one foot, and hop without losing balance	Exhibits excessive swaying (Romberg's sign) and needs to put feet out to keep from falling; cannot stand on one foot or lacks strength to hop
Walking coordination		
• Instruct patient to walk naturally across room; observe patient's balance, arm swing, and gait. Then have patient close eyes and repeat process. • Ask patient to walk heel-to-toe (tandem walk) across room; again observe the balance, arm swing, and gait. **THE CHILD** Observe the child's gait and fine motor coordination during play. Encourage hopping or tandem walking. Note that children under age 5 have a wide, imprecise gait.	Swings arms opposite to movement of legs; first foot fully touches floor as second foot pushes off; with each step, patient shifts weight naturally from one foot to other; maintains balance while doing tandem walk **THE ELDERLY** Elderly patients may have a diminished gait with shuffling or short steps.	Unsteady gait; uncoordinated arm swing; unnatural foot movement with wide steps, shuffling, awkward foot-lifting movements, or staggering; feet may cross in front of one another; cannot maintain balance during tandem walk or cannot do tandem walk **NURSE ALERT** Abnormal Gaits *Dystrophic:* Waddling gait, with legs far apart and weight

ASSESSING CEREBELLAR FUNCTIONING (CONTINUED)

ASSESSMENT TECHNIQUE	NORMAL FINDINGS	DEVIATIONS FROM NORMAL
Walking coordination (continued)		NURSE ALERT (Continued) awkwardly shifted from side to side Dystonic: Nondirectional gait, with jerky movements Steppage: Knee and foot are raised unnecessarily high, then plantar foot is brought to floor with hard, slapping motion.

ASSESSING MOTOR FUNCTION

The nerves for the motor system, like those of the sensory system, originate from the spinal cord and control muscle movement. The following techniques will help you in assessing motor function for your neurologic patient. The only tool required in this assessment is a tape measure.

ASSESSMENT TECHNIQUE	NORMAL FINDINGS	DEVIATIONS FROM NORMAL
RANGE OF MOTION (ROM) HAVE PATIENT PERFORM THESE ROM EXERCISES ON HIS OWN; THEN, PERFORM THEM ON PATIENT.		
Step #1		
• Start with patient's upper body. Have patient relax left arm while you support the right elbow with one hand. Grasp patient's wrist with your other hand and turn his arm in the complete ROM. Repeat process with the right arm.	Can easily relax muscles and has full ROM in all extremities	Muscles exhibit flaccidity, rigidity, jerking motions, or spasticity; patient reports pain; cannot relax muscles and muscles resist movement

ASSESSING MOTOR FUNCTION (CONTINUED)

ASSESSMENT TECHNIQUE	NORMAL FINDINGS	DEVIATIONS FROM NORMAL

RANGE OF MOTION (ROM) (CONTINUED)

- Support patient's left knee and hold the heel with your other hand. Use the same technique as above to check ROM on each leg.
- Grade ROM using this scale: full ROM against gravity, extreme resistance, grade 5; full ROM against gravity, some resistance, 4; full ROM against gravity, no resistance, 3; full ROM with no gravity, 2; slight visible contraction, 1; and no movement, 0.

Step #2

• If ROM results are abnormal, have patient sit on edge of bed with feet dangling and muscles relaxed; hold up both of patient's feet by the heels and then take away your hands.	Legs drop freely and noticeably	Legs are rigid and drop only slightly or not at all

ASSESSING MOTOR FUNCTION *(CONTINUED)*

ASSESSMENT TECHNIQUE	NORMAL FINDINGS	DEVIATIONS FROM NORMAL
OBSERVING THE MOTOR SYSTEM		
• Check patient's muscle strength, size, tone, and involuntary movement. Have patient sit with arms at each side and observe the symmetry of the posture and muscle outlines. • Palpate the muscles for size and consistency. Note any involuntary movements, such as tremor or tics, and any irregular voluntary movements (for example, rapid and jerky movements). Look for any muscle wasting or fasciculations. • Measure patient's muscles in both upper arms, upper thighs, and calves. Compare the measurements for each set of muscles.	Muscles appear to be of equal size and show no signs of involuntary movement; symmetrical posture; muscles in the arms, upper thighs, and calves are same—or very close—in size	Asymmetrical posture while sitting; atrophy of certain muscles or muscles on one side of body; spasticity, flaccidity; twitches or tics; difference in size of muscles when measured
WRIST FLEXIBILITY		
• Tell patient to relax left arm; grasp area just above wrist and shake wrist and hand. Repeat on right wrist.	Wrists move freely	Rigid or spastic movement

ASSESSING MOTOR FUNCTION (CONTINUED)

ASSESSMENT TECHNIQUE	NORMAL FINDINGS	DEVIATIONS FROM NORMAL
Arm drift and arm strength		
Step #1		
• Have patient stand with eyes closed and hold out both arms with palms facing up for 30 seconds.	Can hold this position for 10 seconds with little or no movement in arms	Tries to turn palms down (pronation), lower arms, or bend at elbows; tremor or involuntary movement suggests muscle weakness
Step #2		
• Ask patient (who still has eyes closed) to extend both arms over head with palms facing outward for 30 seconds. • Stand behind patient and tell him to resist your attempts to push his arms back down to the sides.	Can comfortably maintain arms in air with little or no involuntary movement	Arms or hands begin to drift downward; weakness appears on one side; patient cannot resist your attempts to push his arms down
Step #3		
• Ask patient to open eyes and extend right arm. • Instruct patient to resist your efforts to push down on the arm; repeat on left arm.	Comfortably extends arm, holds it in place, and can easily resist your pressure on it	Cannot hold arm out or resist pressure you're applying; tips of shoulder blades may protrude abnormally

ASSESSING MOTOR FUNCTION *(CONTINUED)*

ASSESSMENT TECHNIQUE	NORMAL FINDINGS	DEVIATIONS FROM NORMAL
ELBOW, WRIST, AND HAND FLEXION AND ABDUCTION		

Step #1

- For elbow flexion and extension test, stand at patient's left side; hold patient's upper arm with one hand and wrist with the other. Tell patient to pull the arm toward his body while you pull in the opposite direction. Then exert pressure in the opposite way by having patient extend the elbow while you push back with your hand. Repeat on the other arm. | Can resist counterpressure easily | Muscle weakness (see ROM scale on page 114) or elbow stiffness |

Step #2

- For wrist dorsiflexion test, have patient hold left arm at his side, extend forearm, and make a fist. Put your right hand on the forearm and left hand over the fist, exerting pressure. Repeat on the right wrist. | Easily resists exerted pressure | Weakness in wrist (see ROM scale on page 114) |

Step #3

- To test patient's grip, first hold out your hands with crossed middle and index fingers (middle finger crossed over index). Then ask patient to grab the fingers tightly. | Grip is tight enough to keep you from removing your fingers | Grip is too weak to hold your fingers (see ROM scale on page 114) |

ASSESSING MOTOR FUNCTION (CONTINUED)

ASSESSMENT TECHNIQUE	NORMAL FINDINGS	DEVIATIONS FROM NORMAL

Elbow, wrist, and hand flexion and abduction (CONTINUED)

Step #4

• To test abduction, have patient spread the fingers of one hand while you grip the hand and try to squeeze the fingers back together. Repeat on the other hand.	Exerts enough counterpressure to keep you from closing the hand	Hand is weak under pressure (see ROM scale on page 114)

Step #5

• To test finger flexion and thumb abduction and opposition, have patient hold his left thumb against the left fingertips. Hook your thumb and index finger through the fingers, telling patient to resist your pull. Then try to pry patient's fingers and thumb apart. Repeat on the right hand.	Fingers easily remain together for both tests	Cannot resist pressure on hand (see ROM scale on page 114)

Foot and leg flexibility

• Have patient lie flat on bed; lift his left leg by placing one hand under the knee and the other under the heel; let go of heel while still holding knee. Repeat for other leg.	Leg falls freely and quickly	Leg remains extended or falls rigidly or spastically

ASSESSING MOTOR FUNCTION *(CONTINUED)*

ASSESSMENT TECHNIQUE	NORMAL FINDINGS	DEVIATIONS FROM NORMAL
HIP ABDUCTION AND FLEXION		
• To test hip flexion, instruct patient to lie down; while you press down on his right thigh, have him exert pressure upward. Repeat on left leg. • To test hip abduction, put your hands on either side of patient's knees. Ask patient to try to spread knees against the pressure you exert. • Next, have patient spread legs slightly; place one hand on inside of each knee and ask patient to try to close legs against the pressure you exert.	No difficulty resisting pressure	Muscles are too weak to push back against pressure (see ROM scale on page 114)
LEG AND FOOT FLEXION AND ABDUCTION		
• Have patient remain lying down. Ask him to flex left knee, placing foot flat on bed. Place one of your hands on the knee and the other on the Achilles tendon; instruct patient to resist your pressure to bring the leg down by pulling the foot outward. Repeat on other leg. • Have patient stretch both legs out on bed and then raise one leg. Place one of your hands on the knee and the other on the ankle; tell patient to resist your attempt to push the leg back down. Repeat on other leg.	Can resist all pressure to move legs and feet	Muscles are too weak to resist pressure (see ROM scale on page 114)

ASSESSING MOTOR FUNCTION *(CONTINUED)*

ASSESSMENT TECHNIQUE	NORMAL FINDINGS	DEVIATIONS FROM NORMAL

Leg and foot flexion and abduction *(continued)*

- Next, ask patient to extend legs out straight and point toes upward while you put one hand on the ball of the foot and the other under the ankle. Tell patient to push back with the foot as you push it toward the knee. Repeat on other foot.
- Now, put your hand under patient's ankle again, but this time with your other hand on top of the foot. Tell patient to resist your pressure to pull the foot down. Repeat on other foot.

Assessing the Sensory System

The sensory assessment analyzes the patient's ability to perceive and identify sensations and respond appropriately to stimulation of the extremities. Use the following techniques as a guide to assessing the sensory system of your neurologic patient. Make sure the patient keeps his eyes closed throughout the assessment.

As part of assessing the sensory system, you may also need to check the tendon reflexes, including the deep tendon and superficial tendon reflexes, and to note the pathological reflexes. Use the instructions in the chart that follows as a guide for assessing these reflexes.

𝒯OOLS OF THE TRADE

You'll need the following tools for this assessment: wisp of cotton, cotton-tipped applicator, pin, forceps, tuning fork, two test tubes, hot and cold water, different-sized coins, and paper towel or waxed paper.

ASSESSMENT TECHNIQUES

ASSESSMENT TECHNIQUE	NORMAL FINDINGS	DEVIATIONS FROM NORMAL
Tactile Sensation		
• Touch the skin on patient's right hand lightly with your fingers. Repeat on other hand and the forearms, upper arms, torso, feet, lower legs, and thighs.	Can identify site of sensation and can gauge the lightness or heaviness of the source of touch	Cannot feel fingers or feels the sensation as heavier or lighter than it is

THE CHILD
Allow the child to point to the site being touched rather than naming it. Use this method as needed when testing sensory function.

THE ELDERLY
Consider that, with age, conduction to the peripheral nerves decreases and tactile senses can decrease.

Superficial Pain

• Touch sharp and dull ends of pin or paper clip against patient's upper arm. Maintain even pressure on the touch and occasionally switch from sharp to dull end or dull to sharp end. Assess patient's responses to the different sensations.	Can identify sensations and respond appropriately	Cannot identify different sensations

ASSESSMENT TECHNIQUES *(CONTINUED)*

ASSESSMENT TECHNIQUE	NORMAL FINDINGS	DEVIATIONS FROM NORMAL

Superficial Pain
(continued)

THE CHILD
Don't test the child's superficial pain response with needles.

THE ELDERLY
Some elderly patients have reduced pain sensation.

Temperature Sensitivity

• Fill one test tube with hot water and one with cold water and touch them separately on patient's abdomen for 1 second. Repeat on extremities.	Can identify each sensation and can tell the difference between them	Decreased or absent awareness of hot and cold

---

Sensitivity to Vibration

• Vibrate tuning fork and place it at base of interphalangeal joint of patient's large toe. Assess patient's response. Then stop vibration and again assess response. Repeat on protruding bones of ankles, shins, knees, hips, shoulders, and elbows.	Can identify vibration and knows when it has stopped and can identify pressure from the fork	Cannot identify vibration; can feel only pressure from the fork or has a reduced sense of the vibration

THE ELDERLY
Like tactile senses, vibratory senses can decrease.

ASSESSMENT TECHNIQUES (CONTINUED)

ASSESSMENT TECHNIQUE	NORMAL FINDINGS	DEVIATIONS FROM NORMAL
Deep Pressure Response		
• Have patient lie down and squeeze Achilles tendon on one of his ankles. Repeat on other ankle and on calf and forearm muscles.	Easily identifies the pressure	Cannot feel pressure or can only feel it slightly after prolonged period
Motion and Position Sensitivity		
• Hold patient's index finger between your thumb and index finger and move the finger up and down. Repeat on other hand and on right and left toes, ankles, and knees.	Can feel extremity being moved and can identify direction of movement	Cannot feel movement or cannot identify direction of movement
Cortical and Discriminatory Sensations		
• Use forceps to touch two places at same time on patient's fingers. Then touch only one place and, finally, touch the finger in two places again, increasing the distance between the touches. Repeat on other hand and on arms, torso, and legs.	Can identify number of touches, their location on finger pad, and how many are occurring at once	Cannot properly identify site or number of touches
Point Location		
• Touch patient's hand with cotton-tipped applicator. Repeat on other hand, other extremities, and torso.	Can identify site of sensation	Cannot identify site of sensation or feel sensation

ASSESSMENT TECHNIQUES (CONTINUED)

ASSESSMENT TECHNIQUE	NORMAL FINDINGS	DEVIATIONS FROM NORMAL
Texture Discrimination		
• Place wisp of cotton in patient's hand and ask him to identify it. Repeat process with another texture (for example, paper towel or waxed paper). Repeat entire test on other hand.	Can identify substances and recognize differences between them	Cannot identify substances or feel them
Stereognostic Function		
• Ask patient to identify small objects (for example, various coins or a key) that you place in his palm. Repeat for other hand.	Can easily manipulate and identify common objects	Cannot identify objects or feel them completely
Number Identification		
• Hold onto one of patient's hands; using eraser end of a pencil or your finger, write out a letter or number on the palm. Repeat on other hand.	Can easily identify the number or letter	Cannot identify number or feel it being drawn, or patient can feel sensation in one hand but not in the other
Extinction Phenomenon		
• Use two pins or paper clips to touch symmetrical locations on both of patient's arms simultaneously. Ask patient to identify site of each sensation. Repeat on legs, hands, and feet.	Can feel sensation and can identify its site; feeling is same on both sides of body	Cannot feel sensation or cannot identify its site; can feel sensation on only one side of body

NURSE ALERT

Reflexes, particularly those in the lower extremities, can weaken with age.

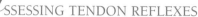
ASSESSING TENDON REFLEXES

- Use a reflex hammer to test the 10 reflexes. Rather than follow a standard for normal and abnormal, use the following scale to grade each reflex response: 4 = hyperactive, 3 = brisk, 2 = normal, 1 = sluggish, and 0 = no reflex.

THE CHILD

When testing pediatric reflexes, remember the following important points:

- Stepping (until age 4 weeks): infant simulates walking when held upright so that both feet touch a flat surface.
- Grasp (until age 3 months): when hand or toes are lightly touched, infant flexes them and tries to grasp.
- Moro (until age 4 months): infant extends and abducts extremities (and may cry) when suddenly startled while lying down.
- Rooting (from ages 3 to 12 months): when cheek is stroked, infant turns head in that direction.

ASSESSING DEEP TENDON REFLEXES

- To test biceps reflex, have patient flex arm while you hold the elbow. Place your thumb over biceps tendon in crook of elbow and strike your thumb with the reflex hammer. Repeat on other arm. Each arm should flex slightly and biceps muscles should contract.
- To test triceps reflex, have patient flex elbow while you hold the wrist. Strike the triceps tendon just above back of elbow. Tendon should contract and extend patient's arm slightly. Repeat on the other arm.
- To test patellar reflex, have patient sit with leg dangling. Strike the patellar tendon just below knee. Knee should extend and cause leg to swing forward. Repeat on other leg.
- To test Achilles tendon reflex, have patient lie down with legs outstretched. Use your hand to hold patient's foot and rotate it outward. Strike the tendon with the reflex hammer and observe for plantar flexion of the ankle. The reaction should be immediate and the muscles should relax quickly after the test.
- To test supinator longus reflex, have patient rest forearm in lap with palm facing down. Use wide end of reflex hammer to strike the radius. Palm should turn upward after the strike. Repeat on other side.

ASSESSING SUPERFICIAL TENDON REFLEXES

- To test abdominal reflex, have patient lie in supine position with arms to side and knees slightly bent. Expose the abdomen and ask patient to exhale. While patient is exhaling, glide a cotton-tipped applicator over the right upper abdomen. The umbilicus should move upward. Repeat on left upper abdomen and on the two sides of the lower abdomen. The umbilicus should move down during assessment of lower abdomen.
- To test cremasteric reflex in male patients, draw the cotton-tipped applicator down the upper part of the inner thigh. The cremasteric muscle should contract and the testicle should rise slightly. Repeat on other side.
- To test plantar reflex on the foot, lightly trace the outer portion of the foot—from the heel up across the ball—with the cotton-tipped applicator. Repeat on other foot. Toes should curl downward.

ASSESSING PATHOLOGICAL REFLEXES

- During test for plantar reflex, if great toe moves forward and other toes separate, patient is showing Babinski's reflex, which indicates presence of neurologic disease. Retest patient for plantar reflex and check for corresponding signs, such as dorsiflexion of ankle and flexion of knee and hip.

NURSE ALERT:
In children up to age 1 year, Babinski's reflex is considered an expected finding; after this age, it can be considered an abnormal finding.

- To assess for ankle clonus reflex, support patient's knee and hold the foot up, pressing toward the knee. The foot should stay in this position with no further movement. Suspect ankle clonus reflex if foot moves back and forth between dorsiflexion and plantar reflex.
- Assess for Brudzinski's sign by having patient lie flat. Ask patient to flex neck forward. Patient should accomplish this comfortably. Pain, resistance, or hip-knee flexion accompanying the position indicates Brudzinski's sign.
- Have patient lie flat and flex one hip and knee. Pain or resistance to this movement indicates Kernig's sign.
- To assess for decorticate posture, observe patient while he is lying flat. Signs of decorticate posture include abnormal flexion of foot, thigh, wrists, forearms, or

lower arms in response to pain; no response to pain; and abnormal eyeball movement when turned side to side.

ASSESSING RELATED SYSTEMS

Below are guidelines for assessing structures and systems related to the nervous system and typical diagnostic tests and procedures used in evaluating the neurologic patient. Tools you'll need for this assessment are a sphygmomanometer and a stethoscope.

Autonomic Nervous System:

Assess the patient for abnormalities or deficits in the following areas:
• Changes in skin color (for example, pallor or cyanosis)
• Perspiration
• Temperature of skin
• Changes in skin or nail quality
• Change in blood pressure with posture change

Neurovascular System:

Assess for normal functioning of the following:
• Blood pressure in each arm
• Brachial pulses
• Carotid pulses
• Temporal artery pulses

Also check for presence of carotid or supraclavicular bruits and for tenderness or nodules at the temporal pulses.

Skull:

Assess for deficits or deformities in size, contour, and prominences. Check for presence of orbital or cranial bruits and for any tenderness on percussion.

Spine:

Assess the vertebral column for possible deformity, tenderness, and bruits and for signs of meningeal or nerve root irritation.

*S*UGGESTED READINGS

Carpenter, A. B., and B. Malcolm. *Core Text of Neuroanatomy.* 4th ed. Baltimore: Williams & Wilkins, 1991.

deGroot, Jack, and Joseph G. Chusid. *Correlative Neuroanatomy.* 21st ed. E. Norwalk, CT: Appleton & Lange, 1991.

DeMyer, William E. *Technique of the Neurologic Examination: A Programmed Text.* 4th ed. New York: McGraw-Hill, 1994.

Way, Christine, and Milena Segatore. "Development and Preliminary Testing of the Neurological Assessment Instrument." *Journal of Neuroscience Nurse* 26.(October 1994): 278–281.

SECTION III: HEAD TRAUMA

$\mathcal{C}$hapter 7: Lacerations and Cerebral Injuries

▽　▽　▽　▽　▽　▽　▽

$\mathcal{I}$NTRODUCTION

SEE TEXT PAGES

Lacerations (deep cuts in the scalp), one of the most common head injuries, are typically not life-threatening and are usually caused by a blunt or sharp force. Lacerations frequently occur in younger children because they are highly active but not well coordinated and their heads are large in proportion to their bodies.

Two types of cerebral injury, concussion and contusion, can seriously damage the brain. A concussion results from a blow to the head or from the brain hitting the inside of the skull because of an acceleration-deceleration force. A contusion is a laceration or bruise across the surface of the brain that alters the structure of the tissue and thus causes neurologic deficits.

$\mathcal{S}$UPPORTING ASSESSMENT DATA

Lacerations:

▼
▼
▼
▼
▼

- To assess the extent of the wound, palpate it carefully, paying particular attention to any puncture wounds, which may have penetrated the brain.
- Usually, the injury will require little more than antiseptic cleaning and suturing.

NURSE ALERT:

The greatest danger from a laceration is profuse bleeding. Keep in mind, however, that a small wound may look much worse than it really is because of the great amount of blood flow. The only benefit to this large blood flow is that infection is rare.

Concussion:

- Actually the effect of a blow to the head; temporarily disrupts the reticular activating system, creating a loss of consciousness, which is the first sign. Another common

sign is short amnesia about the event.
- Other signs and symptoms of concussion include headache, nausea, vomiting, and possibly brief loss of vision and skull fracture.
- Additional signs and symptoms that may occur later with a severe concussion are continued syncopal episodes, coordination deficits, decrease in organizational skills, numbness, tinnitus, and diplopia.
- After concussion, patient requires constant observation, particularly if the period of unconsciousness was greater than 3 minutes. Loss of consciousness for more than 6 hours is considered a cerebral contusion.
- In postconcussion syndrome, the effects of the trauma recur; these effects include continued headaches, episodes of memory loss, syncope, insomnia, restlessness, irritability, and decreased concentration.

Contusion:
- Can be caused by an acceleration-deceleration injury or blunt trauma to the head; does not cause hematoma.
- Most significant sign is loss of consciousness for more than 6 hours.
- Other signs and symptoms: altered level of consciousness, nausea, vomiting, generalized weakness, hemiparesis, visual disturbances, confusion, speech problems, impaired balance, and seizures (in about 5% of patients).
- Contusions to specific areas of the brain each have unique effects.
  - Cortical: neurologic effects are usually related to sight; patient may develop seizures.
  - Brain stem: a potentially life-threatening injury characterized by decreased consciousness; affects cranial nerve function; patient can have bilateral abnormal flexion or extension.
  - Frontal or bitemporal: typically related to a closed-head or nonpenetrating injury; patient is usually restless.
- Patients with signs of contusion must be hospitalized for observation.

*C*hapter 8: Skull Fractures

▽   ▽   ▽   ▽   ▽   ▽   ▽

*I*NTRODUCTION

SEE TEXT PAGES

Skull fractures are common and do not always indicate a brain injury. However, you should closely observe any patient with a skull fracture in case a hematoma develops. Additionally, in most cases, a person with a skull fracture should be admitted to the hospital.

*A*SSESSMENT TECHNIQUES

Begin by examining the patient's skull for bruises, bumps, scalp lacerations, or other defects. Also observe for neurologic changes and decreased alertness.

!

NURSE ALERT:

Take precautions (for example, don't move patient's head unless a spinal neck fracture has been ruled out to avoid worsening fracture and patient's condition) in case the patient has an undiagnosed spinal injury or facial bone fracture.

*T*YPES OF SKULL FRACTURES

- Simple Skull Fracture: Also called a linear or nondisplaced skull fracture, a simple skull fracture is a linear crack in the skull with no bone displacement. It usually results from a blow to the head. They primarily affect the skull. They are difficult to palpate and are best diagnosed with x-ray films.

  Observe the patient carefully for any signs of deteriorated alertness or neurologic deficit. Hospitalize the patient for further observation if the fracture runs across a vascular groove or suture line.

- Depressed Skull Fracture: Depressed skull fracture is an indentation—or depression—in one or several of the bones that form the skull. It is much more likely to cause a brain injury than a simple fracture and may create fragments or splinters of bone.

  Assess the patient for level of consciousness, responsiveness, and quality of respiration. To verify the fracture, palpate the skull and take x-ray films of the area. Assess for injury to the cervical area of the spine and to the mandible and maxilla.

If the fracture is near the sinuses, profuse bleeding may occur; if so, assess further for a possible brain contusion or torn brain tissue. Deeply depressed fractures (beyond 5 mm) require neurosurgery.

Basilar Skull Fracture: Basilar skull fractures occurs at the base of the skull. They are difficult to assess and not easily palpated or seen on x-rays films.

This type of fracture is the most serious because of the potential danger for a ruptured meningeal artery or an epidural hemorrhage (90% of all epidural hemorrhages are caused by a ruptured meningeal artery). They may be visible on a computed tomographic scan or on an x-ray film taken using an open-mouthed (Water's) view.

ASSESSMENT TECHNIQUES

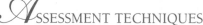

To assess a basilar skull fracture:
- Observe for the following signs:
  - Periorbital ecchymosis (raccoon eyes or owl eyes): bleeding that usually occurs because of an intraorbital root fracture or a cribriform plate fracture.
  - Battle's sign: formation of ecchymosis in the mastoid region; occurs within 12 to 24 hours of the injury.
  - Hematotympanum: blood accumulation behind the tympanic membrane, usually caused by fracture of the temporal bone.
  - Cerebrospinal fluid (CSF) leak: fracture of the temporal bone may cause a CSF leak from the nose (CSF rhinorrhea) or the ear canal (CSF otorrhea). If drainage is clear, place a drop on a dextrose strip; a positive result indicates the presence of CSF because CSF contains glucose. Any blood in the CSF will result in a false-positive for glucose (because blood also contains glucose). If blood is present in the leakage, let some of the fluid drop onto a filter paper; a "halo" or "ring" sign indicates presence of CSF (blood will form an inner circle and the CSF will form a ring around the blood).
- Other signs and symptoms may include a severe headache, a salty taste in throat (from CSF leak), presence of opaque sphenoid sinuses on radiographic examination, and an open fistula at the fracture, causing a CSF leak.

Chapter 9: Classification of Injuries
▽ ▽ ▽ ▽ ▽ ▽ ▽

INTRODUCTION

SEE TEXT PAGES

In the United States, head trauma, the third leading cause of death, is the most common cause of brain damage for people up to age 40.

Traumatic injuries, which usually involve some kind of blow to the head or shearing force on the brain (caused by shaking in infants or motor vehicle accidents), are categorized as focal (specific area of brain is affected) or diffuse (brain cells in many areas are affected). They can also be classified as penetrating and nonpenetrating. In a penetrating injury, the skull is opened or entered; examples include gunshot wounds, stab wounds, or severe fractures from injury. In a nonpenetrating injury, damage is internal, usually caused by a blow to the head or shearing action of brain movement within the skull.

A nonpenetrating injury occurs when trauma forces the brain to move within the skull, hitting the hard bone. Examples include concussions, contusions, and lacerations.

Additionally, both penetrating and nonpenetrating injuries can cause a hemorrhage or hematoma anywhere in the brain. Types include epidural, subdural, subarachnoid, and intracerebral.

ASSESSMENT TECHNIQUES: INITIAL ASSESSMENT

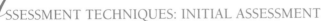

Examine the patient with a head injury as soon as possible. If the patient is unconscious, refer to Section IV, Impaired Consciousness.

NURSE ALERT:

Be aware of pain management medications or any sedation given to brain injury patients. These medications will have a direct effect on your assessment findings.

Additionally, use the following examinations and diagnostic tests to help you make a brief initial assessment and to serve as a basis for later evaluations:
- Cross-table lateral cervical spine radiograph
- Toxicology screen

- Computed tomographic scan
- Pupillary status
- Reflexes

In some circumstances, the following examinations and diagnostic tests may also be useful:
- Skull X-rays
- Magnetic resonance imaging

CONSEQUENCES OF INJURY

The following list of some of the potential effects of head injury will help you assess acute brain injuries and long-term effects of brain injuries. Effects marked with an asterisk have been associated with mild or severe head injuries; patients with mild head injuries may have a lesser degree of a particular effect.

Physical Effects:
- Awkward movements*
- Unsteady gait*
- Paralysis
- Abnormal muscle tone
- Impaired coordination
- Fine motor skill deficits
- Decreased endurance
- Reduced mobility
- Swallowing deficits
- Sensory deficits (visual, olfactory, taste)*
- Speech and communication deficits*
- Facial droop
- Diplopia and blurred vision*

Behavioral Effects:
- Listlessness, lack of motivation*
- Inability to respond to environmental cues
- Violent or suspicious actions*
- Restlessness, easy agitation*
- General intolerance of any kind of stimulation*
- Inattention to issues of personal safety*
- Refusal to eat or obsession with meals*
- Sexually overt actions*
- Using foul language inappropriately*
- Social inappropriateness or lack of social skills*
- Increased inappropriateness toward evening*
- Inability to delay gratification

Psychological Effects:
- Instability (laughing and then immediately crying)*
- Self-absorption*
- Childish, difficult to reason with*
- Looking frightened or dazed*
- Mood swings*
- Denial of deficits
- Changed personality characteristics*

Cognitive Effects:
- Poor or impaired judgment (leads to such behavioral effects as inattention to personal hygiene; not finishing tasks; getting lost; or acting out sexually)*
- Memory deficits*, short attention span
- Confusion, disorientation*
- Personality changes, such as withdrawal and lack of initiative*
- Impaired reading comprehension*
- Difficulty with conversation and word finding*
- Reduced concentration, easy distraction*
- Difficulty integrating information and solving problems
- Impulsive thinking*
- Inflexible thinking*
- Reduced visual and auditory processing
- Decreased speed of information processing
- Impaired ability to plan; inability to follow through with plans

DIFFUSE AXONAL INJURY AND MILD HEAD INJURY

Brain injuries are categorized by the intensity of damage to the neurologic system. Because a head trauma moves the brain within the skull, the axons (communication connectors) may be broken. In mild traumas, axon damage typically occurs in only one place. However, in more severe traumas, diffuse axonal injury (in which microscopic connections are broken in many different parts of the brain) occurs. Long and short term effects of mild head injuries may be difficult to diagnose because the patient's behavior may change in subtle ways. Family members and friends may provide information that can help in the diagnosis.

Chapter 10: Intracranial Hemorrhage

▽ ▽ ▽ ▽ ▽ ▽ ▽

INTRODUCTION

SEE TEXT PAGES

Intracranial bleeding occurs in 30% to 50% of all people who experience traumatic brain injury. Increased pressure from the intracranial hemorrhage—or the hematoma that results from it—can cause potentially life-threatening effects through herniation of the medial temporal lobe and compression of the brain stem. Hemorrhage may occur in any part of the brain; the four types are epidural, subdural, subarachnoid, and intracerebral.

EPIDURAL HEMORRHAGE

The rarest type of intracranial bleeding, an epidural hemorrhage occurs in less than 2% of patients with head injury. It is commonly found in children and the elderly because in these patients, the dura is not firmly attached to the bone and so less severe trauma can result in epidural hemorrhage. About half of all epidural hemorrhages are accompanied by skull fracture. Mortality occurs in 25% to 50% of all cases.

An epidural hemorrhage occurs between the skull and dura mater in the epidural space. The bleeding usually results from a direct blow to the head that causes a tear in the middle meningeal artery or a rupture of the dural sinus.

ASSESSMENT TECHNIQUES

Assessment is usually confirmed with a computed tomographic (CT) scan and an arteriogram. In addition, observe for signs of epidural hemorrhage, which include repeated loss and regaining of consciousness; severe headache; weakness on one side; dilated, fixed pupil on same side as hemorrhage; increased blood pressure; seizures; and slowed heart rate.

SUBDURAL HEMORRHAGE

Subdural hemorrhage, the most common type of intracranial bleeding, results from a severe trauma to the head. The three classes of subdural hemorrhage are acute (lasting 24 to 72 hours), subacute (lasting 72 hours to 10 days), and chronic (lasting more than 10 days).

The bleeding, caused by a torn bridging vein or cortical artery, occurs between the dura mater and arachnoid layer of the meninges. In acute hemorrhaging—usually from a severe injury, such as a high-speed acceleration-deceleration accident—extreme edema can occur, making this condition life-threatening; the mortality rate is over 80%.

ASSESSMENT TECHNIQUES

Observe for the signs and symptoms of acute subdural hemorrhage, which include loss of consciousness, one or both pupils fixed and dilated, positive Babinski's reflex, fever, weakness on one side, and localized hyperreflexia.

THE CHILD

In a child under age 1 year with symptoms of acute subdural hemorrhage, be aware that the child may have been severely shaken in an episode of abuse and proceed accordingly.

To assess for chronic subdural hematoma, look for a history of head trauma, worsening headache, loss of balance, incontinence, change in level of consciousness, signs of dementia, and drowsiness. Any suspicions should be confirmed with a CT scan.

Additionally, keep the following in mind:
- A patient can have a congenital abnormal vessel that can suddenly burst at any age and that can be life-threatening.
- A patient can be free of symptoms at the time of trauma and then develop chronic subdural hemorrhage after a few days, weeks, or even months.
- Elderly and alcoholic patients can develop a subdural hemorrhage without trauma, their symptoms being confused with the onset of dementia.

SUBARACHNOID HEMORRHAGE

A subarachnoid hemorrhage occurs between the arachnoid layer and pia mater of the meninges. The three common causes are severe trauma, severe hypertension, and rupture of a congenital berry aneurysm.

SUPPORTING ASSESSMENT DATA

▼
▼
▼
▼

Signs and symptoms include a history of sudden severe headaches, photophobia, delirium, syncope or coma, generalized tonic-clonic (grand mal) seizures, one or both pupils fixed and/or dilated, weakness on one side, appearance of meningeal irritation, nausea and vomiting, retinal hemorrhage, positive Babinski's reflex, and respiratory difficulties.

INTRACEREBRAL HEMORRHAGE

Intracerebral hemorrhage occurs in the ventricular sinuses or in the brain tissue at any location, usually after a penetrating injury. It may be immediately caused by a laceration, particularly in the basilar region. Intracranial hemorrhage from closed head injury is less common and usually occurs in the frontal or temporal lobes.

SUPPORTING ASSESSMENT DATA

▼
▼
▼

Signs and symptoms include a history of trauma and evidence of basilar injury, weakness on one side, loss of consciousness, and changes in vision.

SUGGESTED READINGS

Carson, Paula. "Investing in the Comeback: Parent's Experience Following Traumatic Brain Injury." *Journal of Neuroscience Nursing* 25 (June 1993): 165–173.

Gennarelli, Thomas A., Howard B. Champion, Wayne S. Copes, and William J. Sacco. "Comparison of Mortality, Morbidity, and Severity of 59,713 Head Injured Patients with 114,447 Patients with Extracranial Injuries." *Journal of Trauma: Injury, Infection, and Critical Care* 37 (December 1994): 962–968.

Mattox, Kenneth L., ed. *Complications of Trauma.* New York: Churchill Livingstone, 1994.

SECTION IV: IMPAIRED CONSCIOUSNESS

Chapter 11: Identifying Levels of Consciousness

▽   ▽   ▽   ▽   ▽   ▽   ▽

INTRODUCTION

SEE TEXT PAGES

One of the first areas you'll assess in a patient with a neurologic disorder or trauma is the level of consciousness (LOC). Patients with acute brain injury usually exhibit a change in their LOC. A patient's LOC can change in a matter of minutes or over many months.

Generally, a conscious individual is someone who is aware of self and surroundings; a decreased LOC is any diminishment in this awareness. The two elements of consciousness are arousal (appearance or state of wakefulness; with decreased LOC, patient may exhibit confusion, delirium, obtundation, stupor, or coma) and content (number and quality of mental functions patient can use).

FUNCTIONING OF CONSCIOUSNESS

Consciousness is controlled by the reticular activating system (RAS).

Dysfunction in the RAS or cerebral hemispheres can affect LOC. Changes in or damage to the RAS may cause more serious deficits in LOC, such as coma. The most serious disruptions to LOC are stupor and coma. In general, LOC is altered by destruction of brain structures and tissue by a lesion, a metabolic disorder, toxic substances, or internal disruptions such as infections resulting in cerebral edema. In some cases, these causes may be life-threatening.

NURSE ALERT

The following changes in LOC can be life-threatening. Changes to tissue structure:
- Abscess
- Edema (increasing intracranial pressure) ⟩
- Hemorrhage
- Aneurysm
- Contusion
- Encephalitis

Metabolic problems:
- Oxygen depletion or shutoff (anoxia)
- Hypoglycemia
- Ischemia
- Vitamin deficiencies (particularly thiamine and niacin)

Internal system failures:
- Organ failure, such as diabetic ketoacidosis, hypertensive or hepatic encephalopathy, and acute adrenal failure
- Fluid or electrolyte imbalance, such as dehydration, acidosis, alkalosis, hypernatremia or hyponatremia, hypermagnesemia or hypomagnesemia, and hypercalcemia or hypocalcemia

Body temperature disruption:
- Hyperthermia
- Hypothermia

Exposure to toxins:
- Use of sedatives or alcohol
- Use of opioids or cocaine
- Exposure to heavy metals (such as lead)
- Exposure to chemicals (such as cyanide, phosphates, and ethylene glycol)

Infections and foreign bodies:
- Meningitis
- Reye's syndrome
- Sepsis

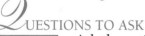

QUESTIONS TO ASK

Ask the patient—or family members or friends if the patient cannot respond—the following questions to assess LOC:

- When did the change in level of arousal occur? (Other changes may include those to the personality, memory, or outward behavior.)
- Was the change sudden?
- Has your condition continued to worsen? If so, how has the deterioration progressed?
- Was there a precipitating event? If so, please describe. Specifically, have you been involved in an accident, recently been exposed to temperature extremes, used drugs or medications of any kind, recently been exposed to a serious infection such as meningitis, recently had dental work or any infections of the ear, sinus, or mastoid?

- Have you experienced any nausea or vomiting? If vomiting occurred, was it projectile and ongoing?
- Have you had any visual disturbances, dizziness, or headaches? If patient had a headache, ask if the pain was severe and if it was diffuse or localized.
- Have you had any abdominal pain, diarrhea, or urinary incontinence?
- Have you had any seizures?
- Have you had a fever?
- Are you sensitive to or have an intolerance to light?
- Do you have any weakness in the back or legs or any progressive weakness?
- If the patient is pregnant, ask if she currently has or previously had pregnancy-induced hypertension.
- Were you possibly exposed to lead?
- Do you have any predisposing conditions or risk factors, such as smoking, sudden life stress, or history of cardiac problems?
- Are you taking any prescription or over-the-counter medications? Which ones, why, how much, and how often?

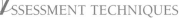

ASSESSMENT TECHNIQUES

The physical assessment of a patient with decreased LOC provides you with objective data about your patient's condition. (See Using the Glasgow Coma Scale.)

Current research focuses on an expanded neurologic assessment instrument that assesses LOC using eight areas of motor, verbal, and brain stem activity. Clinicians are reporting the need for a more complex assessment to improve Glasgow Coma Scale effectiveness in monitoring the patient and predicting outcomes.

USING THE GLASGOW COMA SCALE

A score of 7 or less on this scale indicates that the patient is comatose and experiencing serious neurologic damage. Use the scale for the initial assessment to build a baseline and for subsequent assessments to determine improvement or deterioration.

TEST	RATING
Best motor response	
Obeys simple verbal commands	6
Localizes painful stimulus	5
Flexion withdrawal	4
Abnormal flexion (decorticate rigidity)	3
Abnormal extension (decerebrate rigidity)	2
No motor response	1
Best eye-opening response	
Spontaneous opening	4
Opens on verbal command	3
Opens on painful stimuli	2
No eye response	1
Best verbal response	
Oriented and able to converse	5
Confused but able to respond	4
Inappropriate words or disorganized speech	3
Unintelligible sounds	2
No verbal response	1

USING DERM

You can use the DERM mnemonic, an easy-to-use method to help you remember many of the components involved in assessing LOC.

LETTER (MEANING)	PROCEDURE
D (depth of coma)	• Use verbal and pain stimuli to assess for verbal and motor responses and responses to commands. • Using a normal speaking voice, ask patient to open eyes, move extremities, and answer basic questions about personal identity, time, and place. If patient doesn't respond, raise your voice. If patient still doesn't respond, use a loud noise, such as clapping. • Use painful stimuli after verbal stimuli. Begin by shaking the patient's arm while calling out his name. If patient doesn't respond, apply a pain stimulus (such as pressure to the nail beds) and check motor response. Other appropriate stimuli include pinching the trapezius muscles or grasping the gastrocnemius. • Classify motor responses as purposeful (patient withdraws from pain; may push away source of pain), nonpurposeful (patient slightly moves stimulated extremity, with no attempt to push away source of pain; may slightly contract muscles), or unresponsive (patient does not respond). • Indicate the type of stimulus when documenting the patient's responses; consistency in type of stimuli is recommended. • Check for abnormalities in flexion and extension.

USING DERM (CONTINUED)

LETTER (MEANING)	PROCEDURE
E (eyes)	• Ask patient to open eyes; open the patient's eyes if he doesn't respond. Check pupils for equality and reaction to light. Use assessment techniques for cranial nerve III. Check for ptosis and nystagmus. • Assuming there is no cervical spinal injury, perform oculocephalic and oculovestibular testing.

R (respirations)	• Check patient's respiratory rate, rhythm, and depth. Assess for the cause and signs of abnormal respiration according to the following patterns:
	  - Cheyne-Stokes respiration: controlled by hemispheres in diencephalon; indicated by repeating cycles of hyperpnea, then slowing of respirations to the point of apnea.
	  - Central neurogenic hyperventilation: Controlled by midbrain and pons; indicated by constant, quick hyperpnea.
	  - Apneustic respiration: controlled by pons; indicated by extended inspiratory pauses.
	  - Cluster breathing: controlled by low pons and high medulla; indicated by irregular sequences of breaths and irregular pauses.
	  - Ataxic: controlled by medulla; indicated by respirations with irregular depth and irregular pauses.

M (motor response)	• Check for any abnormal flexion or extension of limbs at rest. • Assess deep tendon reflexes, including Babinski's reflex and posturing reflex. • Assess major muscle groups using a scale from 0 (no function) to 5 (normal), with 1 = slight motion, 2 = movement with no gravity, 3 = can move against gravity, and 4 = weakness.

When using DERM, also do the following:
- Palpate the patient's head for crepitus, a symptom of hematoma or fracture.
- Palpate the abdomen for hepatomegaly as well as any specific areas of tenderness or pain.
- Check the skin for signs of drug use, such as needle marks or tracks. Also, a patient who uses cocaine may have a perforated septum.
- Note if patient has an abnormal breath odor; a sweet smell may indicate a diabetic coma.
- Evaluate heart sounds for widening or narrowing of pulse pressure.
- Monitor blood and urine results, especially for glucose, blood gases, and electrolytes.

Chapter 12: Altered Consciousness

▽ ▽ ▽ ▽ ▽ ▽ ▽

INTRODUCTION

SEE TEXT PAGES

Most comatose patients will emerge from their coma in 2 to 4 weeks. However, some remain in an altered state of consciousness; the three most common states are persistent vegetative state, locked-in syndrome (LIS), and brain death.

PERSISTENT VEGETATIVE STATE

A serious cerebral injury can result in a vegetative state, which can be subacute or chronic. Although patients can emerge from a vegetative state, the state is considered persistent when it lasts beyond 1 month with no sign of emergence (also known as coma vigil or irreversible coma).

In a persistent vegetative state, a patient still maintains the following:
• Vital signs
• Spontaneous respirations
• Sucking, gag, and corneal reflexes
• Periods of wakefulness (though not alertness)
• A sleep-wakefulness cycle
• Occasional open eyes

However, the patient will not exhibit any of the following:
• Orientation to self
• Orientation to environment
• Voluntary actions
• Behavioral responses
• Ability to speak
• Experience of pain

LOCKED-IN SYNDROME

A patient with LIS (also known as de-efferented state, pseudocoma, and ventral pontine or ventral brain stem syndrome) is oriented to self and to the external environment but cannot move or communicate. The voluntary muscles are in a state of paralysis, and in some cases, the patient cannot breathe without mechanical assistance.

In most cases, LIS results from a basilar artery occlusion that causes a brain stem infarct in the ventral pons but leaves the cortical functions intact; it can also result from myasthenia gravis and poliomyelitis.

Manifestations of LIS include:
• Quadriplegia
• Mutism
• Bilateral facial paralysis
• Bilateral tongue paralysis
• Aphasia or dysphasia
• Reduction or loss of horizontal gaze

The areas that usually remain intact are the reticular activating system (making wakefulness and arousal possible)
and cranial nerves III and IV (allowing for eye movements
and eye blinking). The patient's ability to move the eyes is
therefore the only means of communication.

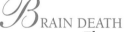
BRAIN DEATH

The concept of brain death has arisen in face of the ability
of modern technology to mechanically sustain vital life
processes such as heart rate and breathing—that is, to use
technology in place of the brain to direct basic functions.

To diagnose brain death, three criteria must be met:
• Absence of basic brain stem reflexes (gag, corneal,
  pharyngeal, oculovestibular, pupillary)
• Absence of cortical function
• Demonstrated irreversibility of this state

The diagnosis of brain death is generally accepted in the
United States if the three criteria listed above are met.
Brain death is considered irreversible if the following are
true:
• Patient does not respond to or withdraw from painful
  stimuli; electroencephalogram is flat.
• The diagnosis represents a disorder capable of causing
  brain death.
• An examination shows loss of brain stem functioning
  and is reproducible.
• Any mitigating factors that could imitate brain death
  (drug overdose or toxicity, hypothermia, shock) have
  been ruled out.
• A full 24 hours has passed without any change in neurologic status.
• A physician conducts the brain apnea test, which
  involves systematic removal of the ventilator from the
  patient and demonstration that the patient is incapable of
  spontaneous respirations.

UGGESTED READINGS

Allison, Malorye. "Predicting Coma Recovery: On the Outside Looking In." *Headlines* 3 (July-August 1992): 2–11.

Connell, Kathleen, Mary Beth Borg, Lynn Cavaliero, Ilana Ross, and Anna Watchmaker. "From Coma to Discharge: The Story of a Roller Coaster Recovery." *Nursing92* 22 (June 1992): 44–50.

Fox, Carol, and Marjorie Lavin. "Vertebral Artery Dissection Resulting in Locked-In Syndrome." *Journal of Neuroscience Nursing* 23 (October 1991): 287–289.

Scherubel, Janet C., and Maureen M. Tess. "Measuring Clinical Confusion in Critically Ill Patients." *Journal of Neuroscience Nursing* 26 (June 1994): 146–150.

*C*hapter 13: Assessment of Intracranial Pressure

▽ ▽ ▽ ▽ ▽ ▽ ▽

*I*NTRODUCTION

SEE TEXT PAGES

Intracranial pressure (ICP), a normal, protective function of the brain, can become problematic when it increases past the point at which the brain structures can balance and process it. Increased ICP can cause severe damage to the brain tissue and, in turn, to neurologic function.

*P*ATHOPHYSIOLOGY

The skull serves as the first layer of protection for the brain; the meninges and cerebrospinal fluid (CSF) cushion the brain and brain structures. Inside the cranial cavity are brain tissue (80%), blood (10%), and CSF (10%). ICP represents the balance maintained by these three components and the combined pressure they exert. If the volume of one of the three components increases, the other two must compensate. Note that CSF pressure greater than 15 mm Hg is life-threatening.

Intracranial pressure also plays a role in cerebral perfusion pressure (CPP), in which brain tissue is perfused. Normal findings for CPP, which is calculated by subtracting ICP from mean arterial pressure, are between 80 and 100 mm Hg. An increase in ICP will produce a decrease in CPP, signaling a decrease in arterial pressure. A drop in CPP to less than 60 mm Hg can mean a sharp decrease in blood flow, raising the risk of cerebral ischemia and infarction.

*C*AUSES OF INCREASED ICP

Any of the following may increase ICP:
- Cerebral lesion expanding the volume of brain tissue; lesion can be caused by trauma, hemorrhage or hematoma, cerebrovascular accident, intracranial tumor, or abscess

- Hepatic or renal encephalopathy
- Infections that block CSF pathways
- Infections, such as meningitis, that prevent CSF reabsorption

Besides neurologic disorders, other conditions and interventions can cause increased ICP in at-risk patients, including:
- Increased blood levels of carbon dioxide
- Decreased oxygen levels
- Suctioning upper respiratory system for longer than 15 seconds
- Valsalva maneuver
- Severe coughing and sneezing
- Positioning that inhibits venous return
- Isometric exercise
- Excessive physical or emotional stimulation

ASSESSMENT TECHNIQUES

Begin your assessment by checking the patient's level of consciousness, particularly level of arousal, interpretation of environmental stimuli, and orientation. Next—and most important—check the patient's pupillary response, including pupillary reactions to light, consensual response, and accommodation. Pupillary responses are governed by the oculomotor nerve, which is often most directly affected by herniation of brain tissue caused by increased ICP.

If ICP continues to increase, bilateral pupillary dilation and fixation may follow; papilledema can also occur, although it is usually seen only with slowly increasing ICP.

Other signs of increasing ICP include:
- Visual disturbances, such as diplopia, blurring, and decreased visual acuity
- Changes in motor function, such as hemiparesis on the opposite side of the lesion
- Decreased arm or leg strength
- Headaches
- Vomiting
- Change in heart rate (bradycardia)
- Changes in blood pressure, particularly Cushing's phenomenon, a critical sign of late-stage increased ICP
- Changes in respirations, from slow to periods of irregular deep and shallow breaths (indicating brain stem compression)

• Changes in temperature, particularly a sudden rise, indicating pressure on the thermoregulatory center

ASSESSING SIGNS AND SYMPTOMS

SIGN	EARLY FINDINGS	LATE FINDINGS
Level of consciousness	Lethargy, restlessness, disorientation	Coma
Headache	Vague complaint	Increased pain
Motor function	Contralateral hemiparesis	Decorticate, decerebrate posturing; flaccid muscles
Vital signs	Stable	Cushing's phenomenon, irregular respirations
Visual changes	Blurring, decreased acuity, diplopia	Can't be assessed
Vomiting	Not present	Projectile (when present)
Temperature	Normal	Elevated
Papilledema	None	May be present
Pupils	Ipsilaterally dilated; slow in reacting to light	Bilaterally dilated, fixed
Brain herniation	Onset, based on pupil responses	Present

*C*hapter 14: Herniation Syndromes
▽ ▽ ▽ ▽ ▽ ▽ ▽

*I*NTRODUCTION

SEE TEXT PAGES

When brain tissue begins to herniate, an extremely dangerous condition, the compensatory system meant to balance
increased intracranial pressure cannot handle the level of
increase and the brain tissue swells, leading to protrusion
and herniation. Increasing herniation is dangerous because
the brain and nerves can shut down against the tremen-
dous pressure. Eventually, pressure against the blood vessels and cranial nerves inhibits their function, and pressure
against the medulla region can compromise the respiratory
and cardiovascular systems.

*P*ATHOPHYSIOLOGY

The intracranial area is divided into three compartments
(the left and right hemispheres and the posterior fossa) by
three rigid membranes: falx cerebri, tentorium cerebelli,
and falx cerebelli. When cerebral edema or a mass, such as
a tumor or hematoma, exerts uneven and forceful pressure
in one compartment of the brain, the cerebral structures
expand into another. Herniation can be either lateral or
downward, depending on the site of the increased pressure.

The three structures most likely to herniate are the cingulate gyrus, uncus of the temporal lobe, and cerebellar ton-
sils. The three types of herniation that correspond to these
structures are cingulate, uncal, and transtentorial. In cingulate herniation, a lesion increases in size, producing pressure that results in movement of falx cerebri. Uncal herniation shifts the temporal lobe laterally, and transtentorial
herniation displaces brain stem tissue downward.

ASSESSMENT TECHNIQUES

TYPE OF HERNIATION	LOOK FOR:
Cingulate	• Slight shift in vital signs and in the earlier symptoms of increased intracranial pressure.

ASSESSMENT TECHNIQUES *(CONTINUED)*

TYPE OF HERNIATION	LOOK FOR:
Uncal	• Ipsilateral pupillary dilation • Paralysis of the eye muscles (ptosis) • Deterioration in energy • Restlessness • Decrease in sensory functions • Contralateral hemiparesis or hemiplegia • Bilateral Babinski's reflex • Respiratory changes (Cheyne-Stokes respirations, hyperpnea, ataxia) • Decerebrate or decorticate posturing
Transtentorial	• Stupor to coma • Cheynes-Stokes respiration • Small, reactive pupils • Gradual loss of vertical gaze • Contralateral hemiplegia • Ipsilateral rigidity to decorticate and decerebrate posturing • Loss of brain stem functioning • Eventually, dilated, fixed pupils; flaccidity; and respiratory arrest

*C*hapter 15: Cerebrovascular Accidents

▽ ▽ ▽ ▽ ▽ ▽ ▽

*I*NTRODUCTION

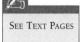

SEE TEXT PAGES

Cerebrovascular accident (CVA), commonly known as a stroke, is an event in which a sudden disruption in the blood supply, and thus oxygen supply, to the central nervous system causes neurologic deficits. CVA is the third leading cause of death in the United States and the leading cause of disability because cutoff of the blood supply to the brain can cause long-term or permanent neurologic damage. CVA can occur at any age, although it is typically associated with the elderly (over age 65); current statistics suggest that about 20% of CVAs affect those under age 65, many of whom are younger than age 40.

Cerebrovascular accident can be classified as ischemic (thrombotic and embolic; 80% of all strokes) or hemorrhagic (intracerebral and subarachnoid; 20% of all strokes). Other types of strokes include transient ischemic attacks (TIAs)—sudden, reversible episodes of neurologic deficit caused by a disruption in the blood supply—and lacunar or small-vessel strokes, which may occur alone or as a continuation of a thrombotic CVA. An episode that lasts more than 24 hours but resolves completely within 48 hours is described as a reversible ischemic neurologic deficit.

*T*YPES OF CVA

Cerebrovascular accidents are classified according to how they develop. However, all CVAs share some basic characteristics:

- They occur after an artery supplying the brain bursts or becomes too clogged to allow blood to flow. Deprived of oxygen from the blood, brain tissue quickly begins to deteriorate and areas of the body controlled by the affected brain cells cannot function properly.
- They typically affect one side of the body more than the other, depending on which side of the brain the event occurred. The effects are related to the hemispheric divisions of the brain: a CVA on the left side generally causes deficits on the right side of the body, and vice versa.

NURSE ALERT:
When assessing a patient with a possible CVA, note on which side the patient is experiencing weakness; the side opposite the weakness is the side on which the CVA has occurred.

- Seizures occur in 8% to 10% of patients with CVAs; in most patients, the initial seizures appear in the first week after the CVA.

CVAS: TYPICAL FINDINGS

TYPE	CAUSES AND ETIOLOGY	FINDINGS
Transient ischemic attack	• Blood flow is temporarily interrupted to a specific area of the brain; possible causes of this interruption are an embolus or atherosclerosis	• Fleeting symptoms; can last from a few minutes to several hours • Carotid and cerebral artery symptoms: hemiplegia, blindness in one eye, cognitive deficits (such as difficulties with speech and momentary confusion) • Vertebrobasilar artery symptoms: dizziness, feelings of numbness, speech disturbances, double vision • Symptoms disappear rapidly; seen as a warning sign of a more serious thrombotic CVA, possibly in a few hours • Can also occur for years before a CVA occurs

CVAS: TYPICAL FINDINGS (*CONTINUED*)

TYPE	CAUSES AND ETIOLOGY	FINDINGS
Thrombotic	• Most common type in patients over age 50; associated with atherosclerosis • Narrowed, clogged cerebral arteries cut off blood supply to the brain; process can occur over many years • Most common sources are embolisms in the middle cerebral artery and occlusions in the cartoid artery	• May take hours or days to develop • May occur during sleep or may be present when the patient first awakens • Usually occur in the large arterial vessels; most common site is the middle cerebral artery • Usually preceded by warning sign of TIAs • Produces various deficits, depending in what section of brain the thrombus occurs; diagnosis may be based on ruling out other types of CVA
Lacunar	• Related to thrombotic CVAs • Small events involving the small blood vessels that may be caused by cerebral edema pressure	• Occur in steps, peaking in a few days • Often occur when patient is asleep or inactive • Onset may be preceded by TIAs • Typically occur in pons
Embolic	• Often results from other cerebrovascular disease, particularly heart disease • Emboli may break off from a thrombus in the heart and pass into the brain via the carotid arteries, causing an occlusion; may also block the middle cerebral artery	• Develop quickly, possibly within 1 to 2 minutes; warning signs are rare (occasionally, a headache) • Usually occur while patient is awake • Embolus may pass through a vessel for only a few minutes, causing temporary symptoms and relatively minor neurologic deficits; may completely resolve in a few days

CVAS: TYPICAL FINDINGS (*CONTINUED*)

TYPE	CAUSES AND ETIOLOGY	FINDINGS
Embolic (*continued*)	• Other sources of embolism include fat buildup within vessels, tumor cells, infection, and clotting caused by such conditions as varicose veins or such procedures as cardiovascular surgery or venous grafts	• Large embolus may lodge in a brain vessel for several hours or may break up, causing smaller clots to lodge in other cerebral vessels • Emboli tend to move peripherally in the brain, creating cortical deficits
Hemorrhagic	Cerebral hemorrhage • Precipitating factors: severe hypertension (most common), ruptured cerebral aneurysm (see Chapter 16, "Aneurysms") or arteriovenous malformation (see Chapter 17, "Arteriovenous Malformations"), or bleeding disorder • Pressure from severe hypertension can rupture an artery, causing bleeding into deep brain tissue, usually at circle of Willis • Blood often cannot clot because of this pressure; thus, bleeding will spread into subarachnoid space, where it will form a clot Intracerebral hemorrhage • Usually occurs deep in the brain in basal ganglia, thalamus, or cerebellum • Displaces cerebral tissue, increasing intracranial pressure	Cerebral hemorrhage: • Generally occurs without warning when patient is awake and active Subarachnoid hemorrhage: • Develops rapidly; may be accompanied by photophobia and cervical stiffness Intracerebral hemorrhage: • Severe hemorrhage can lead to brain stem herniation • Intracranial hemorrhage usually develops over minutes or hours; may be preceded by headache, nausea, and vomiting

SUPPORTING ASSESSMENT DATA

Assessment of CVA includes subjective data collection, general physical examination (with evaluation of vital signs), and thorough neurologic assessment with evaluation for stroke syndromes.

Subjective Data Collection:

Ask the patient (or a family member if the patient's level of consciousness [LOC] is affected) if any of the following have occurred:

- Sudden weakness or numbness of face, arm, and/or leg; weakness will usually occur on one side of the body (note the side)
- Loss of speech, difficulty talking, or difficulty comprehending speech; difficulty writing, calculating numbers, and understanding numbers, words, or pictures
- Sudden onset of severe headache
- Decrease in or loss of vision, especially in one eye
- Alteration of LOC
- Dizziness
- Unsteady gait

Risk Factors:

Assess for risk factors for CVA, as outlined by the American Heart Association and the National Stroke Association:

- Middle to older age
- Race (higher incidence among black women and Chinese)
- Sex (higher incidence among men)
- Heavy smoking
- Excessive alcohol consumption
- High-fat diet (obesity)
- Drug abuse

Health History:

Assess for a history of any of the following conditions that may cause CVA:

- Atherosclerosis (elevated cholesterol level)
- History of TIAs
- History of embolus
- Elevated hematocrit
- AIDS
- Cardiac disease
- Traumatic injury
- Hypertension

- Aneurysm
- Arteriovenous malformation
- Bleeding disorders
- Vasculitis
- Diabetes

Emotional State:

Assess patient's emotional state; symptoms of emotional change after CVA include:
- High reactivity
- Lack of social inhibitions
- Intolerance of stress
- Inappropriate hostility
- Withdrawal, depression
- Social isolation

NURSE ALERT

The following factors are especially important to note with younger patients:

Drug and alcohol use
- Cocaine use: associated with subarachnoid CVA, intracerebral hemorrhage, and cerebral infarction
- Amphetamine use: associated with intracranial hemorrhage (called "speed" hemorrhage)
- Increased alcohol use: linked to hypertension and hemorrhage

Other issues
- Use of oral contraceptives
- Mitral valve prolapse
- Hypercoagulable states, such as sickle cell anemia, protein S disorder, protein G deficiency, antithrombin III deficiency, lupus anticoagulant, and idiopathic thrombocytopenic purpura
- Metabolic disorders, such as homocystinuria

ASSESSMENT TECHNIQUES

Use the following chart as a guideline to performing a physical examination in patients with CVA.

TYPE OF CVA	ASSESSMENT/SIGNS AND SYMPTOMS
Thrombotic Middle cerebral artery syndrome	• Headaches, including location, intensity of pain, length • Hemiparesis and sensory deficits, usually in face rather than extremities • Occasional dysphagia • Aphasia (global) if dominant hemisphere is affected • Cheyne-Stokes respirations • Vasomotor paresis • Inability to move eyes to side of paralysis • Deteriorated consciousness (may lead to coma)
Internal carotid artery syndrome	• Any recurring bouts of blindness or blurring in ipsilateral eye (on side of lesion) • Episodes of contralateral (opposite) weakness in face and extremities; if so, note any complete hemiplegia or sensory loss • Headaches, including location, intensity of pain, length • Hemiparesis and sensory deficits, usually in face rather than extremities • Occasional dysphagia • Aphasia (global) if dominant hemisphere is affected • Cheyne-Stokes respirations • Vasomotor paresis • Inability to move eyes to side of paralysis • Deteriorated consciousness (may lead to coma)
Anterior cerebral artery syndrome	• Incontinence • Sensory deficits in only one leg • Lower-extremity paralysis • Apraxia in extremities on one side • Grasp and suck reflexes present

ASSESSMENT TECHNIQUES *(CONTINUED)*

TYPE OF CVA	ASSESSMENT/SIGNS AND SYMPTOMS
Posterior cerebral artery syndrome	• Homonymous hemianopia (main sign) • Memory deficits • Confusion • Loss of pinprick and touch sensations
Brain stem (Most common cause is Wallenberg's syndrome, which affects lateral medulla)	• Difficulty with muscle coordination • Vertigo • Nausea • Difficulty speaking or swallowing • Loss of facial sensation on ipsilateral side • Loss of sensation in extremities contralateral to site of lesion • Horizontal nystagmus • Miosis, ptosis, anhidrosis (Horner's syndrome) • Brain stem CVAs that occur in pons region cause sensory deficits
Hemorrhagic Cerebellar hemorrhage	• Headaches • Vomiting • Decreased strength in lower extremities • Visual disturbances • Ipsilateral facial weakness
Intracerebral hemorrhage in the putamen	• Headaches • Visual field deficit • Hemiplegia • Cortical deficits • Deviation of eyes away from side of paralysis and toward site of hemorrhage

ASSESSMENT TECHNIQUES *(CONTINUED)*

TYPE OF CVA	ASSESSMENT/SIGNS AND SYMPTOMS
Hemorrhages in pons and thalamic regions	Pons: • Possible hemiplegia • Comatose • Pinpoint pupils • Quadriparesis • No response to ice water caloric test Thalamic: • Possible hemiplegia • Severe sensory deficits • Small, nonreactive pupils
Subarachnoid hemor-rhage	• Headaches • Stiff neck • Decreased LOC • Coma (after the hemorrhage) • Blood leaking into cerebrospinal fluid Can occur at different arterial sites, each with specific symptoms: • Middle cerebral (aphasia) • Posterior communicating (possible palsy of oculomotor nerve [CN III]) • Anterior communicating (possible frontal lobe deficits)
Lacunar Pons lesion	• Risk factors, such as smoking or hyperten-sion • Hemiplegia of face, arm, and leg • Slurred speech and mild weakness in one arm • Ataxia and weakness in one leg
Thalamic lesion	• Risk factors, such as smoking and hyper-tension • Sensory loss in face, arm, and leg

ONGOING ASSESSMENT

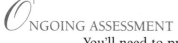

You'll need to provide ongoing assessment and intervention for your CVA patient to help restore circulation to the affected area of the brain and to prevent and manage cardiac complications and increased intracranial pressure (ICP).

Use these guidelines in this assessment:
• Maintain airway patency; inadequate ventilation causes hypoxia and hypercapnia.
• Assess respiration; check for rate, depth, and rhythm. Depressed rate or irregular rhythm are signs of brain stem compression.
• Check heart rate and rhythm; atrial fibrillation is a major risk factor for embolic stroke.
• Monitor blood pressure; previous or current elevated blood pressure may result from cerebral perfusion or a neurologic insult, such as a thrombotic or an embolic stroke. Blood pressure must remain high enough for cerebral perfusion without causing increasing ICP. If blood pressure is lowered, be alert for signs and symptoms of vasospasm.
• Observe for temperature changes; if the hypothalamus is affected, hyperthermia can result.
• Monitor urine output and electrolyte levels; check for endocrine problems such as diabetes insipidus and syndrome of inappropriate antidiuretic hormone secretion.
• Watch for bowel dysfunction; impairment can occur because patient is dehydrated or immobile or has LOC deficits.
• Monitor for seizures to prevent further brain damage.
• Evaluate LOC, which can indicate the state of ICP in your patient; decreased LOC may be an early sign of increased ICP. Assess for these other early and late signs of increased ICP:
  - Early signs: headache, difficulty following commands, restlessness, weakness, confusion, lethargy, drowsiness, slow pupillary response.
  - Later signs: vomiting, respiratory irregularities, loss of gag and swallowing reflexes, hemiplegia, presence of Babinski's reflex, abnormal flexion or extension, ECG abnormalities, increased systolic blood pressure, widening pulse pressure, atrioventricular block.

Chapter 16: Aneurysms
▽ ▽ ▽ ▽ ▽ ▽ ▽

INTRODUCTION

SEE TEXT PAGES

Aneurysms, which involve the blood vessels of the brain, are small, round, saclike enlargements in the wall of the artery that develop because the arterial wall is weak at that particular site. Aneurysms can cause neurologic damage because they rupture and bleed, creating pressure and decreasing oxygen flow. Most aneurysms are less than 1 cm across, although they can increase in size to 5 cm; aneurysms typically occur in people aged 35 to 60. Many people can have aneurysms and never know it; the aneurysms may remain inactive for a lifetime.

PATHOPHYSIOLOGY

The cause of aneurysms is speculative; one suggestion is that they are congenital defects because the wall of the aneurysm is different from that of the arterial wall. Hypertension and polycystic disease have been linked to the presence of aneurysms, although they are not known to be direct causes. However, trauma, especially a shearing force or gunshot wound, can weaken the arterial walls, enabling development of an aneurysm.

TYPES OF ANEURYSMS

There are five types of aneurysms. They include:
- Berry: most common type; named for its stem and neck; probable cause is a defect in the arterial wall; may be linked with polycystic disease.
- Giant (fusiform): related to hypertension; large (at least 3 cm); can compress cerebral tissue and cranial nerves.
- Charcot-Bouchard: also associated with hypertension; a microscopic formation on the basal ganglia or brain stem.
- Traumatic: an injury that can weaken the arterial wall.
- Mycotic: an aneurysmal formation that can develop from the septic emboli of an infection, although this is highly unusual.

ASSESSMENT TECHNIQUES

The majority of cerebral aneurysms occur in the circle of Willis, specifically in the anterior portion. The internal carotid, posterior and anterior communicating, middle cerebral, and anterior cerebral arteries—those most commonly involved in aneurysms—account for 85% of all aneurysms; the remaining 15% develop in the vertebrobasilar system. In almost all cases, however, aneurysms develop at the bifurcation between two arteries; this juncture seems to be a weak area.

Before Onset of Aneurysm:

- Greatest danger of an aneurysm is its dormancy; patients usually don't experience any symptoms until the aneurysm is already occurring.
- Fewer than 50% of patients experience the few warning signs that are known—a nonspecific headache, followed by lethargy, neck pain, and, finally, localization of the headache; some patients also hear a bruit inside their head.
- If the aneurysm is large enough, it may cause some deficits in the optic, oculomotor, or trigeminal nerve functions.
- An aneurysm leaves the dormant stage by either rupturing (tearing or breaking in the wall of the aneurysm from which blood flows) or bleeding (when the wall of the aneurysm does not actually break open but thins enough that blood can seep out).

After Aneurysm Occurs:

The primary symptom of a ruptured or bleeding aneurysm is a powerfully violent headache. Subsequent signs and symptoms, which are related to increased intracranial pressure, are:

- Lowered level of consciousness
- Deficits in oculomotor nerve functions, including visual disturbances
- Vomiting
- Hemiparesis or hemiplegia

If the bleeding comes in contact with the meninges, symptoms of meningeal irritation will occur; these symptoms can include:

- Stiff and painful neck
- Possible increased temperature
- Photophobia
- Blurred vision
- Positive Brudzinki's and Kernig's signs
- Irritability
- Restlessness

*C*hapter 17: Arteriovenous Malformations

▽　▽　▽　▽　▽　▽　▽

*I*NTRODUCTION

SEE TEXT PAGES

An arteriovenous malformation (AVM), like an aneurysm, involves the blood vessels of the brain and can cause damage by rupturing and bleeding or by its size, which in some cases can be very large.

*P*ATHOPHYSIOLOGY

AVMs and aneurysms share some characteristics: both involve blood vessels, are usually not detected unless they become active, and are believed to be congenital, although new research indicates that some AVMs may be caused by head trauma either at birth or later in life.

The differences between AVMs and aneurysms are as follows:
• AVMs are not as common as aneurysms and typically strike men between ages 30 and 40.
• AVMs can affect any site in the central nervous system, although the brain is the most common site.
• AVMs involve both arteries and veins; in an AVM, a combination of veins and arteries are linked incorrectly (see Characteristics of AVMs).

The two main types of cerebral AVMs, classified according to site, are parenchymal (in the parenchyma) and meningeal (in the meningeal tissue). Either type of formation can be fed by one or several arteries. The most common arterial source is the middle cerebral, but the posterior cerebral and thalamic arteries can also be involved.

AVMs can result in hemorrhage, ischemia, hydrocephalus, cardiac decompensation (because of the abnormality of the great vein of Galen—seen in children and infants), compression of cerebral tissue and blood vessels, gliosis, and dysgenesis (interference with normal tissue development).

Characteristics of AVMs

- In a healthy individual, the arteries are connected to the veins through a capillary system. In an AVM, the high-pressure arterial vessels are directly connected with low-pressure venous vessels.
- AVMs are believed to develop congenitally because this connecting capillary system normally forms very early in the gestational period.
- AVMs present a threat because the constant pressure the arteries exert on the veins forces the veins to enlarge to handle the flow and thus increases the size of the lesion; AVMs can become large, complicated clusters of veins and arteries.

NURSE ALERT

As with an aneurysm, a patient with an AVM may not experience any signs and symptoms before the lesion reaches the acute stage. Hemorrhage, the most serious symptom of AVM, can—along with the increase in size—create the following signs and symptoms:

- Throbbing or migraine-like headache
- Seizures (can begin focally and eventually become generalized)
- Fainting
- Dizziness and vertigo
- Motor deficits
- Syncope
- Sensory deficits
- Tingling in extremities
- Aphasia
- Dysarthria
- Hearing bruits (especially in children)
- Visual problems, such as hemianopia
- Confusion

 UPPORTING ASSESSMENT DATA

- Level of consciousness: patient may be disoriented and lethargic.
- Pupillary response: pupils are equal and normal in size, but one may react slowly to light.
- Sensory functions: heightened tactile and temperature sensitivity.
- Motor functions: stiff neck (nuchal rigidity), mild ataxia, hemiparesis, coordination deficits.

- Vital signs: increased temperature, blood pressure, and heart rate; decreased respirations.

A long-term symptom of an AVM is the onset of dementia resulting from chronic ischemia of the frontal lobes; this condition can be preceded by increasing confusion and intellectual deficits.

Statistics suggest that after an AVM has bled, it's likely to bleed again within 4 years. By the time a person with an AVM has reached age 40, there is a 72% likelihood that the formation has bled.

$\mathcal{S}$UGGESTED READINGS

Gold, Diane J., and Mary Mahre. "Endovascular Therapy of Neurovascular Malformations." *Journal of Neuroscience Nursing* 25 (February 1993): 38–44.

Leonard, Anne D., and Susan Newburg. "Cardioembolic Stroke." *Journal of Neuroscience Nursing* 24 (April 1992): 69–77.

Morris, John W., and Vladimir C. Hachinski, eds. *Prevention of Stroke.* New York: Springer-Verlag, 1991.

Rising, Cheryl J. "The Relationship of Selected Nursing Activity to ICP." *Journal of Neuroscience Nursing* 25 (October 1993): 302–303.

SECTION VI: SEIZURES AND EPILEPSY

*C*hapter 18: Seizure Classification and Assessment

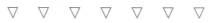

*I*NTRODUCTION

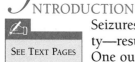

SEE TEXT PAGES

Seizures—sudden, swift bursts of excessive electrical activity—result from changes in electrical patterns in the brain. One out of every 11 persons in the United States will experience at least one seizure. Seizures can arise from a number of conditions, including:

- Epilepsy
- Cerebrovascular accident
- Trauma
- Hypoxia
- Infections
- Lesions from tumors, aneurysms, or arteriovenous malformations
- Fever
- Hypoglycemia or hyperglycemia
- Hyponatremia
- Cocaine use
- Withdrawal from excessive alcohol use
- Inherited traits
- Eclampsia
- Exposure to environmental toxins
- Perinatal injury or congenital and metabolic disorders (children)

Seizures are commonly associated with epilepsy and are one aspect of the disorder; however, an individual does not need to have epilepsy to have a seizure.

*P*ATHOPHYSIOLOGY

Seizures are believed to be caused by any of the following four processes:

- Many cells link together abnormally (hypersynchrony) and fire electrical discharges together (also called storm of activity).
- Cells that inhibit the firing of excitatory cells and the spread of electrical discharges are lost or destroyed.

- An excess of the chemical that signals cells to discharge electrical activity is present.
- Excitatory neurotransmitters upset the neurologic balance that limits the discharge and spread of electrical activity.

SUPPORTING ASSESSMENT DATA

The following are possible symptoms or behavioral changes associated with seizures:
- Shaking or twitching of hands and mouth
- Sensation of "pins and needles"
- Feelings of fear
- Depression
- Body sensations that defy description
- Unusual smells and sounds
- Sudden jerks or nods
- Convulsive movements, typified by sudden rigidity and then relaxation
- Distortion of sensory functions
- Amnesia about seizure event
- Crying
- Vacant stares
- Incontinence
- Aura

Medical History:

You'll need to ascertain if the patient has a history of certain disorders that can frequently cause or be connected to seizures. These disorders include:
- Head trauma with loss of consciousness
- Stroke
- Arteriovenous malformation
- Meningitis
- Encephalitis
- Tumor
- Hyponatremia
- Hypoglycemia or hyperglycemia
- Hypomagnesemia
- Uremia
- Systemic lupus erythematosus
- Thyrotoxicosis
- AIDS

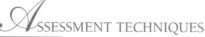

ASSESSMENT TECHNIQUES

To properly assess a patient with seizures, you'll need to note the physical symptoms (the strongest clue to what type of seizure the patient has experienced), ask specific health history questions, and perform a physical examination, including neurologic assessments, electroencephalography, and neuroimaging.

Besides taking vital signs and evaluating function, assess the following:
• Cognitive functions
• Gait and coordination
• Cranial nerve function
• Motor and sensory functions
• Deep tendon reflexes

THE CHILD

Use the following additional guidelines when performing a physical examination on neonates and infants and children:
• For neonates up to age 1 week, assess for neonatal traumatic brain injury and neonatal hypoxic ischemic injury.
• For infants and children, assess for the following:
  - Developmental delays
  - Storage disease (organomegaly)
  - Signs of tuberous sclerosis (adenoma sebaceum)
  - Size differences in the limbs (may indicate early unilateral brain trauma)
  - An enlarged thumbnail or large toenail on one side (may indicate early contralateral cerebral hemisphere injury)
  - History of infection
  - Diagnosis of hypocalcemia
  - Phenylketonuria

THE ELDERLY

In the elderly, assess the carotid artery in the neck region for signs of vascular disorders.

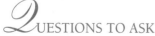

QUESTIONS TO ASK

Obtain a detailed history about the seizure from the patient and any witnesses; include the periods both before and after the seizure as well as during it. Ask the following questions (rationales follow some of the questions):
• Did you experience a loss of consciousness? If so, when?

(Determining if the patient lost consciousness will help you rule out a hypotensive episode from such activity as changing positions too quickly.)
- Are you taking or have you taken any medications? Have you recently made any changes in your use of medications? If so, what medications?
- Have you had any recent significant life stress?
- Do you have a history of drug or alcohol abuse?
- Have you ever experienced an aura? Did you have an aura before this seizure? Did the aura appear suddenly or gradually?
- Describe the sequence of events (patient and witness).
- Were you responsive during the seizure?
- Did you speak or just mumble sounds?
- Did your face color change? Specifically, did it become cyanotic?
- How did your body move? Was it stiff or jerky, or both?
- Did you exhibit automatic movements during the seizure?
- Did you experience either bladder or bowel incontinence during the seizure?
- Did you bite your lips, cheeks, or tongue?
- How long did the seizure last?
- Have similar events occurred before? How frequently?
- After the seizure, were you tired, confused, or depressed?
- Did you experience any postictal paralysis?

TYPES OF SEIZURES

The changes that a seizure causes in a patient's behavior are directly related to where the abnormal electrical charges begin in the brain and how they spread; this process is known as the seizure focus. Seizures are defined according to the seizure focus.

TYPE OF SEIZURE	POSSIBLE SYMPTOMS
Simple (Affect the following areas of function: motor, sensory, autonomic, and psychic)	Motor: • Muscle activity affected • Tonic symptoms: stiff neck, deviation of eyes to one side • Clonic symptoms: jerking movements • One-sided abnormal body movements (jacksonian epilepsy) • Generalized abnormal body movements (secondary generalization)

TYPES OF SEIZURES (CONTINUED)

TYPE OF SEIZURE	POSSIBLE SYMPTOMS
Simple (continued)	Sensory: • Simple hallucinations and illusions, such as buzzing or light flashes • Tactile sensory hallucinations in one limb or extremity • Vestibular involvement
	Autonomic: • Changes in heart rate • Changes in respirations • Pallor • Sweating • Goosebumps • Strange, ill-defined sensations in head, chest, or abdomen • Dilated pupils
	Psychic • Dreamy or foggy state • Decreased attention and cognitive function • Disruption of language and cognitive or memory functions • Spontaneous emotion (for example, sudden happiness, fear, anxiety, depression) • Dissociative phenomena (for example, déjà vu, autoscopy)
Complex	• Preceded by aura • Automatic movements • Staring straight ahead • Wandering • Mindless fidgeting • Lip smacking • Grunts • Repetitions of words and/or phrases • Decreased level of consciousness • Lethargy and confusion after seizure • Amnesia of seizure

TYPES OF SEIZURES (CONTINUED)

TYPE OF SEIZURE	POSSIBLE SYMPTOMS
Secondary generalized	• Possible aura • Spreads from focal to generalized tonic-clonic
Simple absence (formerly petit mal)	• Brief periods of staring and loss of awareness • Usually lasts less than 15 seconds • Immediate return to normal attentiveness • Eye fluttering or blinking • Possibly caused by hyperventilation • Common in children ages 4 to 12 • Amnesia of event
Complex absence	• Staring • Changes in motor functioning, such as sudden hand and mouth movements • Muscle tone changes
Atypical	• Eye blinking • Common in children under age 6 • Frequently found in children with underaverage intelligence • Diagnosis difficult (seizure event may be similar to repetitive motion play)
Tonic-clonic (formerly grand mal or convulsive)	• Loss of consciousness • Stiffening (tonic phase) • Vocalization (cry from air forced through contracted vocal cords) • Jerking of limbs (clonic phase) • Drooling, excessive saliva • Tongue, cheek, or lip biting • Incontinence of bladder or bowel • Amnesia after event • Confusion, lethargy, depression, and deep sleep after event • Onset usually in childhood or young adulthood

TYPES OF SEIZURES (CONTINUED)

TYPE OF SEIZURE	POSSIBLE SYMPTOMS
Tonic	• Stiffening of entire body, arms, or legs • Brief (about 20 seconds) • Common during sleep
Myoclonic	• Jerking postures for a few seconds (clonic) • Brief loss of consciousness possible • Can occur just before sleep • Common in different types of epilepsy
Atonic	• Brief • Sudden loss of muscle tone • Eyelids droop or head nods • Falling • Letting go of anything in hands • Common in childhood
Nonconvulsive	• Ongoing behavioral changes • Continual confusion • No tonic or clonic movements
Convulsive	• Repetitive electrical discharges • Constant systemic and metabolic effects • Potentially life-threatening
Status epilepticus	• Characteristics of both nonconvulsive and convulsive types • Lasts longer than 30 minutes • No recovery of consciousness or function between events • May result from partial or generalized seizure

Chapter 19: Classification and Assessment of Epilepsy

▽   ▽   ▽   ▽   ▽   ▽   ▽

INTRODUCTION

SEE TEXT PAGES

Epilepsy—chronic, although usually intermittent, recurrence of seizure events—results from repeated and abnormal discharge of electrical activity in the cerebral cortex. This discharge can occur in widely varying intervals; some patients have a seizure only every few years. The repetition of the event is the defining characteristic of epilepsy. Epileptic seizures can be partial or generalized.

THE ELDERLY

The onset of epilepsy is typically associated with childhood. However, statistics now indicate that the highest incidence of new-onset epilepsy is among people over age 65. Epilepsy in the elderly may be caused by other conditions common in this age-group, including:

- Tumor
- Trauma
- Dementia
- Infection
- Sustained alcohol abuse
- Cerebrovascular disorders, particularly cerebrovascular accident (CVA)

EPILEPSY CLASSIFICATION

SYNDROME	CHARACTERISTICS
Temporal lobe epilepsy	• Common to both children and adults • Simple, complex, and secondary tonic-clonic seizures • Postictal language deficit when seizures begin in dominant hemisphere

EPILEPSY CLASSIFICATION (CONTINUED)

SYNDROME	CHARACTERISTICS
Reflex epilepsy	• Seizures triggered by external stimuli or internal thoughts • Absence, tonic-clonic, and myoclonic seizures • Photosensitivity (usually to flashing lights) a common cause • Sounds, writing, and arithmetic calculations also seen as cause • Can be outgrown by adulthood
Frontal lobe epilepsy	• Simple and complex partial and secondary generalized seizures • Simple partial seizures originate in motor cortex, causing clonic and tonic movements • Extended electrical discharge through motor cortex causes jacksonian seizure • Symptoms of seizures originating in supplementary motor cortex: contralateral head and eye movement, initial contralateral movement of upper or lower extremities, or ipsilateral movements • Simple partial seizures typified by dizziness, vague symptoms • Complex partial seizures (prefrontal in origin), often of only 1 minute's duration; feature odd, complicated automatisms; may occur in clusters and lead to status epilepticus
Juvenile myoclonic seizure	• Usually adolescent or early adulthood onset • Myoclonic and tonic-clonic seizures in early morning • Chronic, although manageable, condition

EPILEPSY CLASSIFICATION (CONTINUED)

SYNDROME	CHARACTERISTICS
Infantile spasm (West's syndrome)	• Affects children between ages 1 and 4 • Rare; can lead to generalized seizures • Sudden jerks • Stiffening • Winglike flapping of arms • Jackknife seizures (bending forward of body) • May be caused by tuberous sclerosis or injury • Can develop into Lennox-Gastaut syndrome
Febrile seizure	• Affects children between ages 3 months and 5 years • Tonic-clonic symptoms during rising or high fever • Viral infection usually present • Event may last 5 minutes or more • Epilepsy may develop if a family history exists or development is delayed
Benign rolandic	• Affects children between ages 2 and 13 • Stops by age 15 • Controllable by medication • Partial motor or somatosensory symptoms • Family history of epilepsy
Lennox-Gastaut	• Affects children between ages 1 and 6 • Different seizure types (tonic-clonic, myoclonic, tonic, atypical absence) • Seizures usually combined with retardation, slow spike and wave patterns on electroencephalogram • Hard to control, little response to antiepileptic medications • Behavioral problems • Possible causes include trauma, underlying neurologic disorder

ASSESSMENT TECHNIQUES

Assessment for epilepsy involves seeking out the underlying condition causing the syndrome. Follow the same guidelines as in Chapter 18, "Seizure Classification and Assessment"; focus primarily on the following areas:

- Prenatal history
- Developmental history
- Age at seizure onset
- Progression of seizures
- Intervals and frequency
- Precipitating events
- Postictal symptoms
- Injuries associated with seizure events (see Post-traumatic Seizures)

Focus your history taking on the seizure and any precipitating factors as well as on questions specifically concerning the conditions above. Consider the physical changes associated with age, especially in a patient with an abnormal medical history. Pay particular attention to the following conditions:

- Temporary weakness after CVA—can be mistaken for Todd's syndrome
- Aphasia—may hide speech problems caused by seizure
- Cognitive deficits—may be attributed to dementia
- Confusion after seizure—may last for several days, imitating dementia or CVA symptoms

POST-TRAUMATIC SEIZURES

Seizures are a particular concern in patients who have experienced a brain injury. Post-traumatic seizures can occur after the initial symptoms of the injury have become clear or subsided—long after the injury. Epilepsy can develop months or years after the injury.

The two main types of post-traumatic seizures are simple partial (sudden jerking motion) and generalized tonic-clonic (sudden cries, rigidity, and muscle jerking).

Suggested Readings

Kelly William J., ed. *Danger Signs and Symptoms—Clinical Skillbuilders.* Springhouse, PA: Springhouse Corp., 1990.

Laidlaw, John, ed. *A Textbook of Epilepsy.* 4th ed. Edinburgh: Churchill Livingston, 1993.

Legion, Vicki. "Health Education for Self-Management by People with Epilepsy." *Journal of Neuroscience Nursing* 23 (October 1991): 300–305.

Snyder, Mariah. "Revised Epilepsy Stressor Inventory." *Journal of Neuro Science Nursing* 25 (February 1993): 9–13.

Wildrick, Diane. "Neonatal Seizures: The Debate Continues." *Journal of Neuroscience Nursing* 26 (December 1994): 357–363.

*C*hapter 20: Headache Classifications

▽ ▽ ▽ ▽ ▽ ▽ ▽

*I*NTRODUCTION

SEE TEXT PAGES

Headaches, the most common neurologic condition, occur annually in more than 70% of the U.S. population; overall, chronic headaches affect about 50 million people. Although headaches are symptoms of a broader condition, they should also be assessed as a single condition.

The two categories of headaches are primary and secondary. Primary headaches result from an ongoing headache disorder that has no known structural or pathologic cause; the three types are migraine, cluster, and tension or muscle contraction. Secondary headaches are caused by underlying pathologies that can be determined through diagnostic assessment; the four types are referred pain, cranial infections or inflammations, nonmigrainous vascular dilatation, and pressure on intracranial structures.

*P*RIMARY HEADACHES

MIGRAINES

The following chart lists the causes and characteristics of the five types of migraines.

TYPE	CAUSES	CHARACTERISTICS
Classic	• Onset usually in youth (childhood, adolescence, or young adulthood) • Greater incidence among women than men • Family history	• Recurrent • Presence of an aura and unilateral throbbing • Three phases (aura, headache, postheadache) (see The Three Phases of Classic Migraines)

MIGRAINES *(CONTINUED)*

TYPE	CAUSES	CHARACTERISTICS
Common	• Onset can occur at any age • Frequently occurs in reaction to life stresses • Can be related to premenstrual symptoms; may decrease during pregnancy	• May last up to 2 days • Pain is usually throbbing • May be accompanied by nausea, vomiting, and exhaustion • Usually no aura phase • May be accompanied by nasal congestion and fever or chills
Complicated	• Two types: ophthalmoplegic and hemiplegic • In severe pain, underlying pathology may be arteriovenous malformation or other lesion Ophthalmoplegic • Onset usually in young adults • Can begin in middle age, with onset of cardiovascular disease or menopause • Pathology usually involves the oculomotor nerve Hemiplegic • Family history	• Symptoms are especially severe; aura symptoms may continue after headache is gone Ophthalmoplegic • Rare • Extraocular muscle palsies and ptosis on same side as headache • Possible sensory deficits and hemiparesis • Depression, confusion, irritability during headache • Neurologic symptoms may continue after pain stops Hemiplegic • Usually lasts about 1 hour • Hemiplegia or hemiparesis; because of these symptoms, need to rule out more profound pathologies, such as cerebrovascular accidents
Basilar artery	• Onset usually in early adolescence • Occurs because of an obstruction to the blood flow in the basilar artery	• Significant symptoms occur during aura period, including: - Severe visual symptoms, ranging from blurring to blindness - Decreased level of consciousness

MIGRAINES (CONTINUED)

TYPE	CAUSES	CHARACTERISTICS
Basilar artery (continued)		- Vertigo - Confusion - Ataxia - Sudden loss of postural control (drop attacks) • Aural symptoms can occur without a headache following
Status migrainosus	Refer to causes for all other types	• Patient experiences migraines on a constant—even daily—basis

The Three Phases of Classic Migraines

Aura phase:
• Caused by vasoconstriction and decreased serotonin levels; typically lasts for 15 to 30 minutes
• Visual disturbances (for example, spots, flashes of light)
• Possible numbness of face, hands, or lips
• Passing neurologic deficits (brief loss of coordination, brief periods of aphasia and confusion)
• Possible drowsiness
• Aura experience (premonition of attack up to a day in advance characterized by mood change or increased anxiety)

Headache phase:
• Throbbing headache that turns to dull ache
• Usually unilateral pain (may extend to both sides)
• Dilation and distention of cranial arteries
• Possible nausea and vomiting
• Scalp tenderness (from periarterial edema)
• Can last from 4 hours to 2 days

Postheadache phase:
• Aching sensation
• Neck and scalp sensitivity (from muscle contractions)
• Sense of exhaustion
• Movement may extend pain sensations

Cluster Headache

This vascular headache is called "cluster" because it comes on in a series of attacks—or a cluster—over a period of days, weeks, and months and is usually followed by a long remission, perhaps lasting several years. It's also referred to as Horton's headache, histamine cephalalgia, paroxysmal nocturnal cephalalgia, and migrainous neuralgia.

The cluster headache is most commonly found in men; the incidence is five times that for women. Alcohol consumption significantly predisposes a patient to the condition.

Characteristics of the cluster headache include:
- Severe pain often starting 2 to 3 hours into sleep
- Sudden departure of pain, usually after 1/2 to 3 hours
- Extreme unilateral pain (called suicide headache because of intensity)
- Facial flushing, edema, or perspiration
- Miosis or ptosis
- Nasal congestion

Tension Headache

Also called a muscle contraction headache, the tension headache is characterized by a tight, viselike pressure around the head. It may also accompany a migraine in some patients. People most likely to develop tension headaches do work (such as office work) that requires prolonged postures that contract the muscles.

Characteristics of tension headaches can include:
- Gradual onset
- Bilateral pain, difficult to pinpoint
- Frontal lobe predominance
- Pain spreading across head
- Pain in both sides of neck
- Anxiety, nausea, or dizziness in early stages
- Short or long duration
- Scalp tenderness after prolonged headache

Secondary Headaches

Referred Pain Headache

Referred pain headaches are typically caused by pain from trauma, inflammation, or a growth (for example, mass or tumor) in another body region—typically the face or neck. Some sources include:
- Problems in the mouth (such as inflammation of the

gums or tooth abscesses)
- Trauma to, muscles spasms in, or illness of the neck and throat
- Increased intraocular pressure
- Trauma, inflammation, or constant contraction of ocular muscles or eye area
- Infections and allergies involving the sinuses
- Trauma to and infection in the nose and nasal passages
- Infections in the ear

Cranial Infections or Inflammations

This type of pain usually results from a specific disease or disorder in the intracranial or extracranial region, including:
- Arteritis and cellulitis
- Meningitis
- Encephalitis
- Subarachnoid hemorrhage
- Postpneumoencephalographic reaction

Nonmigrainous Vascular Dilatation

With this type of headache, the cranial arteries can dilate—as they would in an actual migraine—in response to environmental toxins, certain drugs, and specific physical disorders, including:
- Use of drugs that dilate the vascular system, such as nitrites and histamines
- Complications from use of hormonal agents, such as oral contraceptives, levonorgestrel (Norplant System), and parenteral hormonal therapy
- Hypertension (headache usually occurs early in the morning)
- Fever or other systemic infection
- Systemic reactions to carbon monoxide poisoning, excessive alcohol consumption, withdrawal from caffeine or nicotine
- Hypoglycemia or other metabolic conditions
- Autonomic hyperreflexia and other acute pressor reactions
- Sudden cerebrovascular insufficiency

Pressure on Intracranial Structures

Headache can be one symptom of increased intracranial pressure. The pressure is usually caused by tumors, hematomas, or abscesses. (See Chapter 13, "Assessment of Intracranial Pressure," and Chapter 14, "Herniation Syndromes.")

Chapter 21: Assessing for Different Headache Types

▽ ▽ ▽ ▽ ▽ ▽ ▽

Introduction

SEE TEXT PAGES

This chapter provides information on how to assess the patient with a headache. A thorough assessment for headache includes the following areas: physical examination; emotional state, affect, and appearance; headache assessment questions; cranial nerve function; motor and sensory function; and reflexes.

Assessment Techniques

Several areas require specific attention during assessment for headache: physical examination, appearance, medication history, headache history, cranial nerve function, diet, skin appearance, and mental and emotional status.

Physical Examination:

Besides performing the basic evaluations as discussed in Section I, ask the patient about and evaluate for the following specific disorders that can cause headaches:
- Hypertension
- Cervical spine abnormalities causing chronic head and neck pain
- Deficits in cerebellar functions, indicating tumors creating increased intracranial pressure
- Distended bladder (common in paraplegic patients)
- Hypothyroidism (evidenced by loss of hair, brittle hair, and dry skin)
- Allergies, which can increase vasomotor activity (particularly seasonal allergies, such as hay fever)
- Anemia
- Local infections in any area of the head
- Temporomandibular joint dysfunction
- Bruits in the neck
- Tenderness over sinus areas
- Family history

Appearance:

Note how the patient presents himself. Keep the following points in mind:

- Many patients who have migraines are careful in their personal appearance and pay great attention to detail. They may come prepared with lists of medications and a written history of their disorder. Depressed patients may have sad facial expressions and a low-key, tired demeanor.
- Other headaches may present obvious physical symptoms, such as Horner's syndrome that accompanies cluster headaches (see Chapter 20, "Headache Classifications"). Neuralgia may also manifest as severe facial pain (for example, in trigeminal neuralgia).

Medication History:

Ask about any medications the patient is taking as well as the dosage and length of time taken. Also ask if the patient has abruptly stopped consuming caffeine-containing foods or beverages or taking any medications. Some medications connected to increased headache symptoms include vasodilators, bronchodilators, and oral contraceptives.

Diet:

Certain foods or substances contained in certain foods have been associated with the onset of migraines, including the following (those foods or substances marked with an asterisk contain tyramine, a substance known to cause headaches):

- Bananas
- Citrus fruits
- Canned figs
- Nuts and peanut butter*
- Avocadoes
- Onions
- Ripened cheeses*
- Pickled or marinated foods, such as herring
- Canned soups*

- Sour cream*
- Chicken livers
- Cured meat products (with nitrites)
- Pork
- Monosodium glutamate
- Aspartame
- Caffeine-containing beverages
- Fresh-baked goods made with yeast
- Chocolate
- Alcoholic beverages
- Vinegar

Tell the patient who can associate any of these foods or substances with the onset of headache to avoid the food or substance.

Skin Appearance:
The following headaches or underlying pathologies can create changes in the skin:
- Hypothyroidism
- Cluster headaches: can produce coarse skin on the face
- Viral infection: for example, postherpetic neuralgia can create lesions on the skin
- Intracranial tumors: may be indicated by the presence of at least five light brown spots
- Intracranial angioma: may be indicated by an angiomata of the skin

Mental and Emotional Status:
Evaluate the patient's mental status by using the tests for cognitive processes described in Chapter 5. Focus particularly on orientation, memory, cognitive skills, and speed of responses. To assess emotional status and identify any stress, ask the patient about the following areas:
- Changes in family relationships or friendships
- Changes in occupation or job status
- Recent vacation or lack of time off
- Recent move
- Oversleeping
- Consistent anxiety
- Current life crisis

Headache History:

Use the following questions and rationales to help pinpoint the source of your patient's headache.

- At what age did the headaches begin? Headaches that start in childhood or up until the 30s are usually vascular, typically migraine. Headaches that occur after the 30s may result from an organic condition (such as a tumor or hematoma), depression, life stress (death or other loss), or trauma.
- Do you have a family history of headaches? This information may be particularly helpful in determining presence of migraine because of the strong family link.
- At what time of day do the headaches occur? Hypertensive headaches usually begin when the patient awakens and continue throughout the day. With cluster headaches, the patient usually awakens with intense pain. Sinus headaches typically start in the morning and worsen as the day progresses.
- How long have you had the headaches? A many-decade history of having headaches may signal a chronic condition. A patient who connects onset with a traumatic event may be experiencing anxiety headaches. However, if onset is sudden and severe, a complete neurologic assessment and diagnostic workup may be necessary; the headaches may be a symptom of an underlying disorder.
- Describe or point to the site of the headaches. Location of the headache can indicate the type of headache. Focal pain on one side of the head could be either a migraine or organic disease; pain that switches sides also is often a migraine. Pain emanating from only the eye can indicate cluster headache, and a "hat band" sensation can signal a muscle contraction headache.
- What is the frequency of the headaches? Women may experience migraines in relation to their menstrual cycle and fluid retention; the headaches often disappear with the onset of menopause. Migraines can also occur in the

first few months of pregnancy. Cluster headaches often are related to change of season. Some patients are relieved from headaches during vacation; others experience headache as soon as they relax. Chronic, ongoing headaches are often the muscle contraction type.

- How long do the headaches last? Migraines can last from a few hours to a few days. Cluster headaches can last from a few minutes to a few hours and usually come on suddenly. Cluster headaches usually recur frequently for a few days or even months before returning to remission. Chronic headache from an organic disorder is continuous and often increases in intensity.
- Describe the pain in as specific terms as possible. Migraines are characterized by intense, pulsating, or throbbing pain, devolving into a dull ache. Cluster headaches are deep and excruciating. Muscle contraction headaches cause a dull, nagging persistent pain.
- Do you have warning signs that a headache is imminent? Migraines are usually preceded by visual changes and, occasionally, paresthesia and a change in the sense of smell.
- Do you have other symptoms that accompany the headache? Patients with cluster headaches may also experience ptosis and constriction of the pupil (Horner's syndrome), tearing, facial flushing or blanching, or perspiration on the face. Migraines can be accompanied by nausea, vomiting, photophobia, and focal neurologic deficits. An intracranial disorder could cause diplopia and unilateral tinnitus. (Compare the described headache types against the patient's symptoms for further reference.)
- Are your sleeping patterns disrupted by the headaches? Migraines often awaken the patient, but sleep generally provides relief. Cluster headaches typically have their onset during sleep, often making falling back to sleep impossible. Patients who experience headache as a symptom of depression usually have no trouble sleeping; patients with headache as a result of anxiety may have difficulty falling asleep.

Cranial Nerve Function:

Assessing the cranial nerves can indicate underlying disorders that may be causing headaches. Below are some findings common to specific cranial nerves:

- Olfactory: a tumor can interrupt the sense of smell
- Optic: touching both eyes can indicate a difference in pressure. Optic atrophy, hemorrhage, papilledema, or exudates can indicate diabetes, hypertension, or brain lesion.
- Oculomotor and trochlear: sudden pain behind the eye can signal an aneurysm. One-sided pupil enlargement can indicate oculomotor nerve compression.
- Abducens: brain lesions can paralyze this nerve on one side.
- Trigeminal: assess this nerve for evidence of trigeminal neuralgia.
- Facial: tests can indicate palsy, residual stroke symptoms, and brain lesion. Signs and symptoms of brain lesions include loss of tearing, loss of taste on anterior two thirds of the tongue, facial weakness or paralysis, and hyperacusis.
- Auditory: unilateral tinnitus and deafness may indicate acoustic neuroma.
- The remaining cranial nerves are not generally associated with headaches.

MOTOR, SENSORY, AND REFLEX FUNCTIONS

Perform assessments of these functions if you obtain evidence of an underlying disorder. Motor, sensory, and reflex assessments can indicate brain lesions, aneurysms, or effects of a cerebrovascular accident, tumor, or hematoma.

SUGGESTED READINGS

Diamond, Seymour. "Head Pain Clinical Symposia." Summit, NJ: Ciba Pharmaceutical Division, Ciba Geigy Corp., 1994, vol 46, no. 3.

Gallagher, R. Michael, ed. *Drug Therapy for Headaches.* New York: Marcel Dekker, Inc., 1991.

Goadsby, Peter J., ed. *Current Opinion in Neurology* 7 (June 1994): 255–282.

Chapter 22: Classification and Assessment of Brain Tumors

▽ ▽ ▽ ▽ ▽ ▽ ▽

INTRODUCTION

SEE TEXT PAGES

Central nervous system tumors result from abnormal growth of the neuroglia or a metastatic growth from a tumor elsewhere in the body.

Central nervous system tumors are classified according to several different criteria.

CLASSIFICATIONS AND CHARACTERISTICS

CLASSIFICATION	CHARACTERISTICS
Age of patient	• CNS tumors occur most commonly in childhood and late middle age. • Typical age ranges are birth to 6 years and over age 45. • Statistically, tumors are more common in children than in adults. • Brain tumors in children are typically found in the infratentorial region.
Primary or secondary	• Primary tumors originate in the CNS. • Secondary tumors have metastasized to the CNS from primary tumors in other parts of the body, usually the GI system, genitourinary tract, lungs, or breasts.
Benign or malignant	• These terms have different meanings for tumors found in the CNS than for those found in the rest of the body: a CNS tumor may not be cancerous, for example, but its location within the brain may make it as deadly as any malignant tumor.

CLASSIFICATIONS AND CHARACTERISTICS *(CONTINUED)*

CLASSIFICATION	CHARACTERISTICS
Benign or malignant *(continued)*	• Benign: not seriously invasive into interior portions of brain; slow growing and easily differentiated from other brain tissue; does not cause serious neurologic deficit; is easily accessible to surgery, which also will not cause serious deficit • Malignant: can be malignant because of makeup or location; invasive and uncontained, with many narrow projections into tissue, making surgery difficult; malignant cells are often difficult to distinguish from normal cells; presence of tumor can cause neurologic deficit, as can its surgical removal because of the complicated structure of the growth; most tumors are categorized as malignant because of their cell structure

Location	• Neurologic deficits caused by a tumor can indicate its location in brain (for spinal cord locations, see Chapter 23, "Classification and Assessment of Spinal Tumors").
	 • The following increasingly specific categories are used to identify the site of brain tumors:
	   - Intra-axial tumors (within central neuraxis)—found in cerebral hemispheres, brain stem, and cerebellum
	   - Extra-axial tumors (outside central neuraxis)—found in meninges, cranial nerves, and pituitary gland
	   - Supratentorial (above tentorium)—found in cerebral hemispheres
	   - Infratentorial (below tentorum)—found in cerebellum and brain stem
	 • Tumors are also identified according to neurologic deficits, which can indicate which specific lobe of the brain is affected.

CLASSIFICATIONS AND CHARACTERISTICS (CONTINUED)

CLASSIFICATION	CHARACTERISTICS
Basic structure (histologic origin)	• Primary CNS tumors are organized histologically according to their general site. This order, created by the World Health Organization in 1979 and generally used by health professionals, includes gliomas (primary intracranial brain tumors that develop from glial cells [neuroepithelial tissue] and are usually invasive), tumors from other brain structures, congenital tumors, and cancerous tumors (see chart below).

CHARACTERISTICS AND SIGNS AND SYMPTOMS

This chart outlines each type of glioma, tumor from other brain structures, congenital tumor, and cancerous tumor.

TYPE OF TUMOR	CHARACTERISTICS	SIGNS AND SYMPTOMS
Gliomas		
Astrocytoma	• Slow-growing; invasive; develops in astrocytes (support tissue for neurons and capillaries); can develop anywhere in brain or spinal cord • Accounts for between 20% and 40% of all intracranial tumors in adults and 30% in children	• Neurologic deficits arise from tumor site • In children, can affect the optic nerve, causing dimness of vision, blindness, and optic atrophy • Grades I and II can effect the cerebellar region, causing sensory loss, gaze disorders, cerebellar dysfunction, facial paralysis, and hemiplegia
Glioblastoma	• Is believed to develop from mature astrocytes and usually arises in cerebral hemispheres • Highly invasive	• Seizures • Changes in cerebral functioning • Specific deficits indicate tumor site

CHARACTERISTICS AND SIGNS AND SYMPTOMS (CONTINUED)

TYPE OF TUMOR	CHARACTERISTICS	SIGNS AND SYMPTOMS
Glioblastoma (continued)	• Often has multiple foci of origin and creates areas of necrosis and hemorrhage, which typically arise in frontal lobe • Accounts for about 30% of all intracranial tumors in adults • Higher incidence in men than in women • Usually occurs later in life • Graded III and IV	
Oligodendro-glioma	• Develops from oligoden-drites (cells for myelin sheath) • Usually arises in cerebral hemispheres, often in frontal lobe or some-times in ventricles • Very invasive with well-defined, globular mass • Slow-growing; often includes calcification • Typically affects people between ages 20 and 40 • Accounts for about 5% of all intracranial tumors	• Specific frontal lobe deficits indicate tumor site • Seizures are first sign in 50% of all patients
Ependymoma	• Develops from ependy-mal cells (lining of choroid plexus and ven-tricular system) • Can arise directly in cere-bral hemisphere or in roof or floor of fourth ventricle, making it hard to remove	• Seizures • Sudden rise in intracra-nial pressure (ICP) • Decreased level of con-sciousness • Changes in vital signs with increase in blood pressure • Pupillary changes • Hemiplegia • Cerebellar dysfunction • Sensory deficits

CHARACTERISTICS AND SIGNS AND SYMPTOMS *(CONTINUED)*

TYPE OF TUMOR	CHARACTERISTICS	SIGNS AND SYMPTOMS
Ependymoma *(continued)*	• Constricts flow of cere-brospinal fluid • Can be either fast- or slow-growing • Benign • Accounts for about 6% of all intracranial tumors • Most common in children	
Medulloblastoma	• Develops from embryonic cells • Usually arises in back of fourth ventricle • Well-defined; fast-growing • Accounts for about 1% of all intracranial tumors • Most common in children	• Squinting • Visual disturbances • Increased ICP • Cerebellar dysfunction, such as loss of coordination
Neurilemoma	• Develops from Schwann cells • Usually arises in cranial nerves (particularly affects vestibular control of cranial nerve VIII) • Slow-growing and benign but often in inaccessible area • Accounts for about 4% of all intracranial tumors • Dizziness • Tinnitus • Vertigo • Hearing loss	• Can enlarge to cause hydrocephalus, loss of coordination, and sensory deficits in cranial nerves V, VII, IX, and X

Tumors from other brain structures

Meningioma	• Develops within and outside of meningeal layers, particularly near venous sinuses	• Neurologic deficits from brain tissue compression • Site indicated by type of deficit

CHARACTERISTICS AND SIGNS AND SYMPTOMS *(CONTINUED)*

TYPE OF TUMOR	CHARACTERISTICS	SIGNS AND SYMPTOMS
Meningioma *(continued)*	• Benign and well-defined • Highly vascular • Compresses other structures and tissue; may erode into skull • Slow-growing • Accounts for 15% of all tumors • Common in women over age 50	
Pituitary tumor	• Develops within pituitary gland, arising in anterior lobe; may extend to third ventricle • Parasellar tumors can crowd gland • May be secreting or nonsecreting • Slow-growing • Accounts for 8% to 12% of all intracranial tumors • Common in older adults	• Headache • Paresis of extraocular muscles • Endocrine disorders (Cushing's syndrome, prolactin-secreting adenoma, growth hormone–secreting adenoma, all with their attendant symptoms) • Visual disorders
Hypothalamic tumor	• Develops within the hypothalamus • Can cause hyperthermia, malignant hyperthermia, or hypothermia	• Increased heat production, possibly decreased cardiac output, heat exhaustion or heatstroke from hyperthermia • Increased oxygen consumption • Tense muscle fasciculations and rigid masseter muscles • Possibly renal failure in malignant hyperthermia • Severe failure of thermoregulation leads to hypothermia, decreased body temperature, and decreased blood pressure

CHARACTERISTICS AND SIGNS AND SYMPTOMS *(CONTINUED)*

TYPE OF TUMOR	CHARACTERISTICS	SIGNS AND SYMPTOMS
Congenital tumors		
Pineal tumor	• Usually arises near pineal gland from residual cells of fetal development • Appears in several types (germinoma, pinealoma, teratoma) • Well defined • Contains cystic areas that can contain cartilage, bone, teeth, and hair • Tends to recur because of nature of fetal cell tissue • Accounts for 1% of intracranial tumors • Most common in people ages 20 to 30; more common in men than in women	• Increased ICP from obstruction of cerebral aqueduct and third ventricle • Melatonin in pinealoma can inhibit sexual development
Craniopharyngioma	• Develops from squamous cells located in or near pituitary • Benign; solidly defined; slow-growing • Can depress anterior pituitary function when located near pituitary stalk • Can also fill third ventricle • Can put pressure on basal ganglia, brain stem, or optic chiasm • Can recur because of nature of fetal cell tissue • Accounts for about 4% of all intracranial tumors • Most common in children and in those aged 30 to 40	• Pituitary and hypothalamic deficits • Visual deficits • Increased ICP • Endocrine function may still be impaired after surgery

CHARACTERISTICS AND SIGNS AND SYMPTOMS (*CONTINUED*)

TYPE OF TUMOR	CHARACTERISTICS	SIGNS AND SYMPTOMS
Dermoid and epidermoid cysts	• Different types that develop from ectodermal layer • Typically arise on bones of skull but can arise elsewhere in brain • Account for (with craniopharyngioma and pineal tumors) about 4% of all intracranial tumors	• Deficits depend on location of cysts
Angioma	• Blood vessel tumor arising from arteriovenous malformation (hemangioma) or embryonic vascular tissue (hemangioblastoma) • Usually located near vertebral column or skull and involves dura • Benign; slow-growing • Irregular, with network-like appearance • Can cause compression in brain and hemorrhage • Accounts for 6% of all intracranial tumors • Most common in females	• Dizziness • One-sided ataxia • Increased ICP • Symptoms of hemorrhage

CHARACTERISTICS AND SIGNS AND SYMPTOMS (CONTINUED)

TYPE OF TUMOR	CHARACTERISTICS	SIGNS AND SYMPTOMS
Cancerous tumors		
Metastatic tumors	• Develop in any part of CNS; often single or multiple growths in subarachnoid space • Result from malignant cells that spread through blood from cancer sites in lungs, GI system, kidneys, prostate, or breasts • Usually well defined • Account for about 10% of CNS tumors • Occur in about 35% of all cancer patients	• Depend on site of growths • Increased ICP
Malignant melanomas	• Usually located in cerebral hemispheres • Highly malignant with poor prognosis	• More than five cafe au lait skin lesions
Primary cerebral lymphomas	• Develop in brain stem, cerebral hemispheres, or cerebellum • Also known as non-Hodgkin's lymphoma • May be either multifocal or monofocal • Can present as a glioblastoma • Rare, but incidence is increasing because of rise in immunodeficiency disorders (particularly AIDS)	• Neurologic deficits • Personality changes and behavioral changes • Apathy • Confusion • Focal signs indicating site of lesion • Appear on computed tomographic scan

ASSESSMENT TECHNIQUES

Begin your assessment with a thorough evaluation of the patient's symptoms. In particular, focus on the following symptoms:

- Headaches
- Seizures
- Nausea and vomiting
- Signs and symptoms of increased ICP
- Cognitive deficits
- Memory deficits
- Expressive aphasia
- Visual changes
- Motor deficits
- Sensory deficits
- Changes in pupillary function
- Loss of bladder and bowel control
- Changes in level of consciousness

The first four signs and symptoms (headache, seizures, nausea and vomiting, and increased ICP) are the most important early manifestations of a brain tumor. About one third of all tumor patients have headaches; up to one half have seizure activity. Both headache and seizures can be accompanied by nausea and vomiting.

Papilledema, which is present in up to 75% of all patients, is a common manifestation of increased ICP. (See Chapter 13, "Assessment of Intracranial Pressure.") Be sure to perform a complete assessment for increased ICP.

You'll also need to identify possible tumor locations based on the patient's signs and symptoms. The chart below provides signs and symptoms for various tumor sites.

VARIOUS TUMOR SITES: SIGNS AND SYMPTOMS

TUMOR SITE	SIGNS AND SYMPTOMS
Frontal lobes	• Cognitive deficits • Memory deficits • Judgment impairments • Emotional instability • Personality changes • Loss of bowel and bladder control • Expressive aphasia • Muscle weakness

VARIOUS TUMOR SITES: SIGNS AND SYMPTOMS *(CONTINUED)*

TUMOR SITE	SIGNS AND SYMPTOMS
Frontal lobes *(continued)*	• Paralysis • Deficits in deep tendon reflexes • Positive Babinski's sign • Papilledema
Cerebellum	• Loss of balance • Gait disturbances • Nystagmus • Loss of coordination • Action tremor • Deficits in deep tendon reflexes • Seizures • Changes in vital signs
Parietal lobes	• Deficits or loss in all sensation (see Chapter 4, "Anatomy and Physiology Review," and Chapter 6, "Objective Data Collection," for more information on sensory assessment)
Occipital lobes	• Deficits in visual field • Perceptual deficits • Hallucinations
Temporal lobes	• Memory loss • Hearing deficits • Receptive aphasia • Hallucinations • Visual field deficits
Pituitary	• Visual changes • Paralysis of extraocular muscles • Hormonal dysfunctions (Cushing's syndrome, hypopituitarism, gigantism, acromegaly)
Hypothalamus	• Changes in water balance • Changes in sleep patterns • Changes in appetite • Fat and carbohydrate metabolism changes • Changes in sexual behavior

VARIOUS TUMOR SITES: SIGNS AND SYMPTOMS (*CONTINUED*)

TUMOR SITE	SIGNS AND SYMPTOMS
Midbrain (rare)	• Cerebral aqueduct occlusion • Paralysis of upward gaze (quadrigeminal plate involvement) • Cerebellar deficits (red nucleus involvement) • Ptosis and light reflex deficits (later stages)
Brain stem	• Vomiting • Lower cranial nerve deficits • Cerebellar deficits • Dysphagia • Sensory deficits • Corticospinal deficits • Sudden death (from pressure on cardiorespiratory center)
Ventricles (lateral and third)	• Headache • Vomiting • Symptoms of rapid ICP increase • Relief obtained by shifting head, changing position of tumor
Ventricle (fourth)	• Headache • Vomiting • Neck and head rigidity • Gag and swallowing reflex deficits • Sudden death (pressure on cardiorespiratory centers)

QUESTIONS TO ASK

During the interview, ask questions about and make observations in the following areas:
• Sleep disturbances
• Sensory and perceptual alterations
• Feelings of hopelessness
• Heightened feelings of anxiety
• Changes in ability to perform daily tasks

*C*hapter 23: Classification and Assessment of Spinal Tumors

▽　▽　▽　▽　▽　▽　▽

*I*NTRODUCTION

Spinal cord tumors, which are less common than brain tumors, account for 0.5% to 1% of all tumors and are one-tenth the number of brain tumors.

*C*LASSIFICATION

These tumors can appear anywhere on the spinal cord, with 30% occurring in the cervical area, 50% in the thoracic area, and 20% in the lumbosacral area. Like brain tumors, spinal cord tumors can be primary (arising from spinal cord cells and structures) or secondary (metastatic).

The two categories of spinal cord tumors are intradural and extradural.

Intradural tumors include intramedullary and extramedullary tumors:
- Intramedullary—originate within the spinal cord; are typically gliomas; signs and symptoms include radicular pain, tenderness, weakness, and loss of joint and vibration sense associated with Brown-Séquard syndrome.
- Extramedullary—originate within the dura or outside the cord; typically neurofibromas, meningiomas, and dermoid and epidermoid tumors; signs and symptoms, which tend to be less easy to pinpoint, include diffuse pain, segmented sensory loss, muscle atrophy, and reflex deficits.

Extradural tumors include metastatic lesions, primary sarcomas, chordomas, neurofibromas, and meningiomas (rare). The most significant symptom that accompanies an advance in development of a spinal tumor is increased intracranial pressure. Such an increase typically causes papilledema, either because of tumor pressure or because of increased protein in cerebrospinal fluid (CSF). (Protein levels increase under normal conditions to signal a need for increased CSF volume.) A syringomyelic syndrome (an intramedullary cyst) may develop, causing chronic, degenerative symptoms, such as pain, weakness, and spasticity. This, however, is not a tumor.

SIGNS AND SYMPTOMS

SIGN OR SYMPTOM	CHARACTERISTICS
Pain	• Most common symptom • Either local, radicular, or medullary referred pain • Patient feels local pain over tumor site, particularly when any kind of pressure (even from movement) is exerted • Patient may feel greater pain after a sudden movement or when lying down because these actions stretch the nerves • Radicular pain can vary in intensity but is often severe; intraspinal pressure from the tumor on the nerve roots directs pain to the region controlled by that nerve • Patient experiences medullary referred pain in peripheral areas, often on both sides; sensation may be of a bursting or burning pain and is often mistaken as a symptom of other disorders, such as appendicitis, angina, or gallbladder problems

Motor deficits	• Symptoms in early stages of tumor development (typically fatigue, weakness, and heavy feelings in extremities) are vague and often easily overlooked
	• Later symptoms that involve the corticospinal tracts can include:
	  - Clumsiness
	  - Spasticity
	  - Paresis
	  - Clonus
	  - Exaggerated deep tendon reflexes
	  - Babinski's reflex
	• Later symptoms that involve the roots of the peripheral nerves can include:
	  - Diminished deep tendon reflexes

SIGNS AND SYMPTOMS *(CONTINUED)*

SIGN OR SYMPTOM	CHARACTERISTICS
Motor deficits *(continued)*	- Extremely diminished muscle tone (hypotonia) - Flaccid paralysis - Muscle fasciculations - Muscle atrophy
Sensory deficits	• Develop because of compression of the tumor • Early symptoms may include paresthesia and numbness; later symptoms may be lateral or unilateral • General lateral symptoms include deficits in pain and temperature sensation and deficits in vibration and proprioception awareness • General unilateral symptoms include ipsilateral spastic weakness, loss of sense of vibration, and loss of sense of joint position
Sphincter dysfunction	• Tumors that bilaterally compress the spinal cord can affect bladder and bowel control • Symptoms of bladder dysfunction as they increase include: - Urgency - Difficulty urinating - Retention - Incontinence • Generally, bladder dysfunction precedes bowel dysfunction; symptoms of bowel dysfunction include constipation and paralytic ileus

Assessment Techniques

Neurologic testing, clinical observations, interview questions, and diagnostic testing rule out other disorders and pinpoint the site, type, and extent of the tumor.

Neurologic Tests

The following neurologic assessment tests are used in diagnosing a spinal tumor:
- Cranial nerve assessment
- Motor assessment (including respiratory difficulty)
- Sensory assessment
- Assessment of deep and superficial reflexes; tests that elicit pathologic reflexes

Clinical Assessment for Location

Below are tumor sites along the spinal cord and their corresponding signs and symptoms.
- Cervical—C4 and above:
  - Occipital headache
  - Stiff neck
  - Respiratory difficulty
  - Atrophy of shoulder and neck muscles
  - Dysphagia
  - Dysarthria
  - Vertigo
  - Quadriparesis
  - Sensory deficits (in area that presents weakness)
  - Possible sacral sparing (Tumors in this area are especially dangerous because of possible involvement of the diaphragm and subsequent respiratory failure.)
- Cervical—below C4:
  - Pain in shoulders, arms, and hands
  - Atrophy of muscles in areas above
  - Muscle fasciculations
  - Paresthesia without pain
  - Horner's syndrome

- Thoracic:
  - Tenderness at tumor site
  - Pain in chest or back
  - Spastic paresis in lower extremities
  - Most effects to sensory system
  - Band of hyperesthesia at tumor site
  - Sphincter dysfunction
  - Beevor's sign
  - Positive Babinski's reflex

NURSE ALERT

Metastatic tumors are most likely to develop in the thoracic region. Sensory assessment is particularly important for this region; motor dysfunctions tend to be minor.

- Lumbosacral:
  - Pain in lower extremities and lower back
  - Spasticity and paresis in one leg and then the other
  - Atrophy to particular muscle groups
  - Diminished reflexes
  - Loss of bladder control

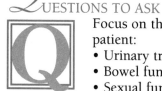

*Q*UESTIONS TO ASK

Focus on the following areas in the interview with your patient:
- Urinary tract function
- Bowel function
- Sexual function

*S*UGGESTED READINGS

Albright, A. Leland. "Pediatric Brain Tumors." *CA—A Cancer Journal for Clinicians* 43 (September–October 1993): 272–288.

Baron, Mary C. "Advances in the Care of Children with Brain Tumors." *Journal of Neuroscience Nursing* 23 (February 1991): 39–43.

Bonilla, Mary Ann, and Nai-Kong Cheung. "Clinical Progress in Neuroblastoma." *Cancer Investigation* 12, no. 6 (1994): 644–653.

DeAngelis, Lisa M. "Management of Brain Metostases." *Cancer Investigation* 12 (March 1995): 156–165.

Laws, Jr., Edward R., and Thapar Kamal. "Brain Tumors." *CA—A Cancer Journal for Clinicians* 43 (September–October 1993): 263–271.

Schiffer, Darude. *Brain Tumors Pathology and Its Biological Correlates.* Berlin: Springer-Verlag, 1993.

Chapter 24: Classification and Assessment of Injuries

▽ ▽ ▽ ▽ ▽ ▽ ▽

INTRODUCTION

SEE TEXT PAGES

Between 7,000 and 12,000 individuals in the United States sustain injuries to the spine in the course of a year; 82% are men. About 80% of injuries occur in individuals under age 40 and 50% occur in those aged 15 to 25.

Besides effects from the actual injuries, patients who have experienced this kind of trauma are at risk for an infarct because of damage to the blood vessels.

TYPES OF INJURIES

Spinal cord injuries can occur to the vertebrae alone, to the vertebrae and spinal cord, or to the soft tissue of the spinal cord (see Soft Tissue Injuries). The greatest risk of these injuries is paralysis below the site of damage to particular nerves.

Quadriplegia (also known as tetraplegia) can result from severe damage to the cervical area of the spinal cord; paraplegia can result from severe damage to the lumbar region. Injuries that affect only the vertebrae are least likely to cause permanent paralysis. However, the presence of a broken vertebral bone is always considered dangerous to the spinal cord.

Other injuries can occur to the neck that do not necessarily involve the spinal cord. The two most common are fractures of the larynx and penetrating wounds. A fractured larynx usually results from a distraction injury or a blunt impact of the neck against the steering wheel of a vehicle. Base your assessment on the presence of a contusion, respiratory stridor, hoarseness, or a cough with bleeding (hemoptysis).

A penetrating wound, usually caused by a knife or bullet, is evident by obvious signs, such as bleeding, swelling, evidence of airway obstruction, shock, hemothorax, and hypovolemia. In addition, deficits may occur in the brain and spinal cord from loss of circulation.

MECHANISMS OF SPINAL TRAUMA

Trauma to the vertebral column and spinal cord can be caused by dislocations of the bone (subluxations), fractures, and penetrating wounds. The mechanisms that cause these injuries are listed in this chart.

MECHANISM	CHARACTERISTICS
Hyperextension	• Head is forced backward, snapping the spine beyond its normal range of motion • Causes whiplash in less severe cases but can tear anterior longitudinal ligaments, stretch the spinal cord, and cause hemorrhage • Accounts for 93% of all spinal trauma • Can be caused by water sports (such as diving), rear-end motor vehicle accidents, and falls in which a person hits directly on the chin
Hyperflexion	• Head is forced beyond its normal range of motion by force of an impact (usually a front-end vehicle collision) that flexes the spine forward, backward, or laterally or causes the head to overrotate, turning beyond normal limits • Posterior longitudinal ligaments can tear, increasing risk of bone displacement
Axial loading or vertical compression	• Blunt force compresses spine, causing damage to spinal structure and possibly bone fragmentation into soft tissue of the cord • Can be caused by blow to head, hard fall onto end of spine or the feet, or compression force to both top and bottom of spine at once
Distraction	• Vertebrae are pulled out of alignment and spinal cord is stretched, possibly causing rupture • Commonly seen after a suicide attempt by hanging

MECHANISMS OF SPINAL TRAUMA *(CONTINUED)*

MECHANISM	CHARACTERISTICS
Penetrating wound	• Sharp injury from a knife blade, bullet, or projectile during an accident • Can penetrate soft tissue directly without injuring the vertebrae

*S*UPPORTING ASSESSMENT DATA

▼ The earliest indications of a spinal injury are:
▼ • Pain in the back or neck
▼ • Numbness or paralysis in extremities
▼ • Unusual position of head or neck
▼ • Bulging in spinal cord

*C*LASSIFYING FRACTURES

Fractures of the vertebral column are classified as follows:
• Simple fractures (does not usually affect alignment or compression; usually found at facets, pedicles, or spinous or transverse process)
• Compression fracture (anterior compression usually caused by hyperflexion injury but may not compress into spinal cord; also known as a wedge injury)
• Burst fracture (shattering of bone, with fragments often pushed into spinal cord; usually results from axial injury)
• Teardrop fracture (fragment of bone breaks off vertebral column, possibly lodging in spinal cord)
• Jefferson fracture (the ring of the first cervical vertebrae [C1] bursts after axial loading; injury does not necessarily affect the cord but can cause death if it penetrates the spinal cord at this location)
• Odontoid fracture (three types of fracture that occur at the C2 level; a dislocation of one vertebra overriding another, usually causing a ligament injury, a partial dislocation of one vertebra, or a fracture through the arch of C2 [known as hangman's fracture]; these injuries are not usually life-threatening or seriously damaging)
• Atlanto-occipital dislocations (an all-or-nothing injury in which the atlas tears away from the occipital bone; either death can result or no neurologic damage can occur)

Also consider vertebral injuries as fracture-dislocations if bone is both fractured and dislocated (as in the teardrop fracture).

Two other categories of fracture are stable and unstable. Injuries are stable if the structures that provide support (the ligaments and some part of the vertebral column) are still intact. Injuries are unstable if there is severe ligament damage and, in most cases, if there is significant damage to the bone.

CLASSIFYING SPINAL CORD INJURIES

Vertebral column injury with spinal cord injury is common because of the close and fragile relationship between the bony vertebral column and delicate spinal cord. The spinal cord can also be damaged because of injury to other support structures. Spinal cord damage can be caused by:
- Transection (severing of the cord that can be complete or incomplete)
- Contusion (bruising that can cause bleeding and edema, resulting in compression of the cord)
- Arterial damage (injury to the posterior or anterior spinal arteries can cut off nourishment to the cord, potentially causing permanent deficits from ischemia or necrosis)
- Systemic and hemodynamic changes (blood flow can decrease because of loss of autoregulation; changes in blood flow then can cause ischemia; lactic acid accumulation can cause an increase in vasoconstriction and vasospasm, also leading to ischemia)

Spinal cord injuries can be further classified as complete, incomplete, or nerve root.
- Complete (involves loss of sensory function, voluntary motor function below the level of damage, and a loss of sense of the body position (proprioception); occurs more infrequently than incomplete injury and typically results in quadriplegia or paraplegia)
- Incomplete (spinal cord retains some function, depending on the site and size of the lesion; sensation remains in perineal region; three syndromes can result—central cord, Brown-Séquard, and anterior cord [see Chapter 25, "Spinal Cord Syndromes and Complications"])
- Nerve root (affects the motor and sensory function in a particular nerve root)

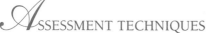

ASSESSMENT TECHNIQUES

Early Assessment: Early nursing observations provide information about the patient's status, including:

- Airway management (ensure airway patency and check for presence of edema and foreign bodies; blind nasotracheal intubation is the intubation of choice).

NURSE ALERT

Never move or try to straighten a spinal deformity without a physician present—the patient's respiratory system might become compromised or further damage to and possibly paralysis of the spinal cord could result. When possible in an emergency setting, don't remove any headgear, such as a motorcycle or football helmet.

- Ability to breathe (assess respiratory rate, rhythm, and depth of breaths as well as for tracheal damage. Injuries to specific cervical nerves can damage the accessory muscles for breathing or the diaphragm: lesions to C3, C4, or C5 can cause paralysis of the diaphragm; lesions to C2 through C8 can paralyze the intercostal muscles; and lesions to T1 through T11 can paralyze the abdominal muscles).
- Circulation (damage caused by hemorrhage and neurogenic shock can affect vital circulatory functions; internal hemorrhage may be difficult to determine if patient has deficits that may inhibit sensory and motor function; these areas require frequent neurologic assessment. Internal hemorrhage requires a computed tomographic scan of the abdominal area).

NURSE ALERT

Neurogenic shock, the loss of vasomotor tone and deficits in autonomic function, is characterized by hypotension and bradycardia, with the skin staying warm and dry. Symptoms of bradycardia include vagal stimulation, hypothermia, and hypoxia.

- Neurologic status (the two areas of greatest immediate concern are level of consciousness and gross deficits. Note whether the patient is alert and the level of his or her responsiveness; observe for any obvious motor or sensory deficits.)
- Physical status (assess for signs of injury, such as contusions and wounds; evaluate the patient's back, using the logroll technique; and check the spine for signs of pain,

edema, or deformity. Neurologic deficits can increase if edema or hematoma are present in the spinal cord; hematoma is particularly dangerous in the posterior pharyngeal region. Assess the patient's body temperature frequently for signs of hyperthermia or hypothermia.)

Secondary Assessment: After stabilizing the patient, assess for the following:
• Injuries (assess the bones of the skull and face for injury).
• Pain (back or neck pain is a clear indication of some kind of dysfunction, although reporting pain depends on the patient having an adequate level of consciousness. Use of drugs and alcohol, stress from trauma, and pain from any other injury can keep the patient from feeling pain; therefore, do not consider absence of pain as an indication that no injury has occurred).
• Cerebrospinal fluid (CSF) leakage (if a penetrating injury is apparent, assess for a CSF leak).
• Sensory deficits (assess for cranial nerve function, particularly sensation to touch and pain and any visual disturbances; use a dermatome map to identify the nerves involved).
• Motor deficits (assess motor strength in all extremities; check for spasms, paresthesia, and paralysis).
• Reflexes (assess deep and superficial reflexes and note presence of pathologic reflexes. Also check for the presence of priapism, the anal wink, and the bulbocavernosus reflex. Test the anal wink by pricking the area near the anus with a pin to elicit a contraction from the anal sphincter; no reaction indicates spinal cord involvement. Test the bulbocavernosus reflex by placing one finger in the patient's rectum while compressing the clitoris or glans or, as required, pulling on a Foley catheter; the anal sphincter should contract).

SOFT TISSUE INJURIES

Disk herniation, although not life-threatening, can cause chronic pain, disability, and limitations. Herniation can occur because of degenerative illness or injury and can be either acute or slow-developing because of posture or occupational stresses.

PATHOPHYSIOLOGY

The soft center (nucleus pulposus) ruptures, putting pressure on the spinal nerves and causing pain. The disk ruptures by pushing through the circular ligament (anulus fibrosus) that usually holds it in place. Disks in the lumbar and upper sacral regions are particularly at risk for rupturing because of their instability in the vertebral column; they are not attached to a major body structure such as the ribs.

Symptoms of herniated disk include:
• Pain
• Numbness or tingling
• Urinary or bowel dysfunction

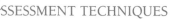

SSESSMENT TECHNIQUES

Assessment includes a review of possible symptoms, a history (including interview questions about onset and possible stressors or injury that might have caused the problem), and imaging, such as magnetic resonance imaging, to determine the site and extent of the problem.

Chapter 25: Spinal Cord Syndromes and Complications

▽ ▽ ▽ ▽ ▽ ▽ ▽

INTRODUCTION

SEE TEXT PAGES

This chapter covers the syndromes and complications caused by spinal cord injuries.

The four main conditions associated with incomplete spinal cord injury are:
- Brown-Séquard syndrome: one side of the spinal cord becomes damaged, usually because of a tumor, penetrating injury, fracture that has affected the cord, or rotational injury. As a result, specific motor and sensory functions are affected—the patient loses proprioception and motor function ipsilaterally and loses pain and temperature sensation contralaterally.
- Central cord syndrome: the center of the cord is damaged, usually by a hyperextension injury that creates a hemorrhage; the center of the cord swells, causing a loss of blood flow. The main symptom is quadriparesis that affects the arms more than the legs because they are controlled by the center of the cord.
- Anterior cord syndrome: results from acute compression of the anterior spinal artery or a herniated disk. The patient experiences sudden and total paralysis below the lesion, including loss of pain and sensation. However, proprioception, which is governed by the dorsal column, remains intact, as do the sensations of vibration and light touch.
- Posterior cord syndrome: results from cervical hyperextension below the level of injury and is characterized by loss of proprioception and sensation to light touch.

COMPLICATIONS

COMPLICATION	CHARACTERISTICS
Pulmonary conditions	• Present most serious threat to patient • Paralysis of the diaphragm or accessory muscles can lead to infection; hypoventilation can cause atelectasis • Pulmonary embolism can occur suddenly, even in patients who have begun to stabilize

COMPLICATIONS (*CONTINUED*)

COMPLICATION	CHARACTERISTICS
Pulmonary conditions (*continued*)	• Pressure on calf muscle, increased coagulability of blood, and loss of skeletal muscle pump can lead to deep vein thrombosis
Orthostatic hypotension	• Usually occurs in the critical and early stages of recovery • Vascular problems can cause feelings of light-headedness, which can develop into syncope, bradycardia, and asystole • Can be caused by loss of skeletal muscle pump and deficits in sympathetic nervous system control over blood vessels
Autonomic dysreflexia	• Also called hyperreflexia • Usually occurs in rehabilitative stage (although it may occur in the acute period) • A noxious stimulus (such as bladder distention, bowel impaction, tight clothing, a blocked indwelling catheter, or lumpy bedclothes) can cause the sympathetic nervous system to release catecholamines, resulting in vasoconstriction • Inhibitory messages sent by the parasympathetic nervous system to decrease blood pressure can't pass through the spinal cord obstruction; therefore, the body experiences two different reactions above and below the point of injury (congestion, headache, and flushed skin above the injury and cold skin below it) • To compensate, vagal stimulation brings on bradycardia to lower blood pressure and cardiac output; however, this is not usually enough to lower hypertension • Patient becomes increasingly at risk for complications of high blood pressure, including heart attack, subarachnoid hemorrhage, and cerebrovascular accident

COMPLICATIONS (CONTINUED)

COMPLICATION	CHARACTERISTICS
GI dysfunction	• Injury typically causes loss of bowel function (patients can't tell when bowel is full and can't aid in evacuation); guard against fecal impaction because of potential autonomic dysreflexia • GI bleeding from body's response to stress
Genitourinary dysfunction	• If bladder becomes atonic, patient won't be able to void urine voluntarily or spontaneously • Patient may begin voiding urine spontaneously after spinal shock is over
Skin integrity	• Patient is at risk for infection, pressure ulcers, and irritants below the point of injury, where sensation is gone • Assess patient's skin regularly for signs of breakdown • Assess nutritional intake

$\mathcal{S}$UGGESTED READINGS

Reich, Steven M., and Jerome M Cotler. "Mechanisms and Patterns of Spinal Cord Injuries." *Trauma Quarterly* 9 (Winter 1993): 7–28.

Sarkar, Soumitra, Corinne Peek, and Jess F. Parker. "Fatal Injuries in Motorcycle Riders According to Helmet Use." *Journal of Trauma: Injury, Infection, and Critical Care* 38, no. 2 (1995): 242–245.

Velmahos, Degiannis, K. Hart, I. Souter, and R. Saadia. "Changing Profiles in Spinal Cord Injuries and Risk Factors Influencing Recovery After Penetrating Injuries." *The Journal of Trauma: Injury, Infection, and Critical Care* 38, no. 3 (1995): 334–337.

*C*hapter 26: Degenerative Diseases

▽　▽　▽　▽　▽　▽　▽

*I*NTRODUCTION

SEE TEXT PAGES

This chapter provides a short description as well as signs and symptoms and brief assessment tips for some of the most common degenerative disorders.

*A*LZHEIMER'S DISEASE

Alzheimer's disease, an organic and progressive brain syndrome that creates profound cognitive deficits and is one of the most significant causes of dementia, occurs most commonly in individuals over age 65 and affects about 5% to 10% of the population. However, the disease also afflicts those as young as age 45.

*S*UPPORTING ASSESSMENT DATA

▲ Physical Findings:

The signs and symptoms of Alzheimer's disease advance in three stages:

- Stage one: characterized by forgetfulness, declining interest in people and surroundings, depression, anxiety, uncertainty, and declining competence in performing work tasks; may take 2 to 4 years to develop.
- Stage two: characterized by increase in memory loss, changes in personality (such as growing irritability and increasingly embarrassing behavior in social situations), night wandering, signs of aphasia, delusions, and inability to manage activities of daily living and household responsibilities; may develop over 2 to 12 years.
- Stage three: characterized by inability to communicate, inability to recognize family members, seizures, incontinence, and inability to walk; may develop over the course of a year and is often followed by death from aspiration pneumonia.

▲ Health History:

Typically, Alzheimer's disease is detected during the second stage. Risk factors include a family history of the disease, a history of myocardial infarction, or a history of head injury.

ASSESSMENT TECHNIQUES

Assessment includes noting the signs and symptoms, performing a neurologic evaluation, and obtaining a magnetic resonance imaging or a computed tomographic scan to detect cerebral atrophy and an electroencephalogram to indicate irregularities in and slowing of brain rhythms. Definitive diagnosis requires a brain biopsy to determine the presence of senile plaques and the identification of levels of choline acetyltransferase, an enzyme involved in development of acetylcholine, which is needed for memory formation.

To assess mental status, evaluate the patient's visual-spatial relations, recent and remote memory, ability to perform numerical calculations, and performance on the Mini-Mental State Examination.

MULTIPLE SCLEROSIS

Multiple sclerosis (MS), a progressive disease that typically affects young adults, involves the slow demyelination of the white matter in the brain and spinal cord. It's characterized by relapsing—and then remitting—attacks of neurologic dysfunction that can occur anywhere in the CNS and can worsen over time. Signs and symptoms of the attacks depend on what area of the nervous system is being affected during the episode. No cure exists for MS; treatment includes management of symptoms and prevention of progressive complications.

SUPPORTING ASSESSMENT DATA

▲ Physical Findings:

The signs and symptoms of MS advance from early to later stages. The time frames for each stage vary according to a patient's condition, thus leading to difficulty in diagnosis because of the wide range of fluctuating symptoms.

- Early stage: characterized by visual abnormalities (particularly optic neuritis), nystagmus, vertigo, ataxia, limb weakness, bladder dysfunction, impotence, shocklike tingling paresthesia radiating from neck to extremities, mood swings, and irritability; symptoms may be difficult to form together into a diagnosis.
- Later stages: characterized by pain, loss of hearing, increasing weakness and spasticity, depression, memory loss, confusion, swallowing difficulties, paralysis, and dementia.

▲ Health History:
Diagnosis involves piecing together a history of relapsing and remitting episodes of neurologic deficit. A definitive recent history includes two or more attacks lasting at least 1 day and occurring at least 1 month apart. A familial history of the disease, Uhthoff phenomenon (also known as the Nor Bath test), worsening symptoms during exposure to heat, and abnormal reflexes contribute to the diagnosis. Additionally, the patient may exhibit Lhermitte's sign (upon flexion of neck, patient experiences electric or shocklike paresthesias that travel from the neck down the arms and legs bilaterally, indicating involvement of dorsal roots of spinal cord posterior columns).

AMYOTROPHIC LATERAL SCLEROSIS
Also known as Lou Gehrig's disease, amyotrophic lateral sclerosis is a wasting disease of the muscles that destroys the motor cells in the gray horns of the spinal cord and degenerates the pyramidal tracts. It progresses rapidly, usually causing death within 3 years, and is three times as common in men as in women.

SUPPORTING ASSESSMENT DATA
▲ Physical Findings:
Look for the following early signs and symptoms:
• Weakness in the hands, often manifesting as increasing clumsiness
• Increasing weakness of muscles in the upper extremities (particularly in the shoulders and upper arms), leading to wasting and atrophy
• Later affect in muscles in the lower extremities; usually cramp and feel heavy and fatigued

Other signs and symptoms include:
• Muscle spasticity and fasciculations
• General fatigue
• Dysarthria and dysphagia (if speech, chewing, and swallowing muscles are affected)

▲ Health History:
• Assess the signs and symptoms and perform a neurologic assessment.
• No definitive tests exist, but an electromyelogram can detect muscle fibrillations (which indicate denervation and muscle wasting).

- Test for elevated levels of serum creatine kinase, which indicate muscle tissue breakdown.

MYASTHENIA GRAVIS

Myasthenia gravis, a progressive disease characterized by muscle weakness that stems from a myoneural junction defect, affects young adults—usually between ages 20 and 30—and occurs at least twice as often in women as in men.

SUPPORTING ASSESSMENT DATA

▲ Physical Findings:

Generally, myasthenia gravis shows muscle group weakness that is exacerbated at the end of the day. The disease is categorized according to degree of severity:

- Ocular—mild symptoms involving ocular muscles alone or ptosis and diplopia; usually remits spontaneously
- Generalized (mild)—mild symptoms begin with ocular muscles and extend to skeletal and bulbar muscles; very slow onset and low rate of mortality
- Generalized (moderate)—begins with ocular muscles and more rapidly extends to bulbar and skeletal muscles, with more severe effects; can restrict independent activities, but still has a low mortality rate
- Generalized (acute fulminating)—swift involvement of skeletal and bulbar muscles and respiratory system, leading to rapid deterioration and high mortality rate
- Generalized (late severe)—deterioration occurs slowly or suddenly 2 years or more after ocular or generalized symptoms, with high mortality rate

▲ Health History:

Assessment for myasthenia gravis includes the following:

- Degree of muscle group weakness
- Tensilon test—myasthenia gravis patients show an immediate, although brief, improvement in muscle tone after injection of the drug
- Electromyographic studies—can identify the myoneural junction deficit
- Serum antibody test for acetylcholine receptors—elevated in almost all myasthenia gravis patients
- Chest X-rays—can identify presence of a thymoma

PARKINSON'S DISEASE

Parkinson's disease, a motor functioning disorder caused by degenerating neurons in the basal ganglia, typically affects the elderly. Symptoms of the disease often go undiagnosed for a long time because they so closely mimic changes that occur with aging.

SUPPORTING ASSESSMENT DATA

▲ Physical Findings:

Below are the primary and secondary signs and symptoms of Parkinson's disease:

- Primary—motor dysfunction, including resting tremor (called "pill-rolling" when present in hands), rigid muscles, bradykinesia (slowed movement, lack of spontaneous movement), changes in posture and gait (stooped posture; gait disturbances, from slow movement to uncontrollable forward propulsion), stiff trunk movements
- Secondary—visual deficits, expressionless (masklike) face, monotone voice, reduction in fine motor control (increasing clumsiness, difficulty with handwriting), general weakness that may lead to patient being bedridden and immobile, muscle fatigue, autonomic symptoms (drooling, constipation, dysphasia, perspiration, oily skin)

▲ Health History:

Assessment includes noting signs and symptoms, testing motor and sensory systems, and asking questions about changes in functioning.

HUNTINGTON'S DISEASE

This slow-developing inherited disorder affects motor and sensory functions and emotional state. The child of a carrier of the gene for Huntington's disease has a 50% chance of developing the disorder. Symptoms do not usually appear until age 35, although they can appear in childhood or old age. The illness is fatal, but patients with active symptoms can live from 16 to 40 years.

SUPPORTING ASSESSMENT DATA

▲ Physical Findings:

- Early symptoms include clumsiness, bradykinesia, falling, depression, apathy, aggression, feelings of confusion, and mild involuntary movements (chorea) involving distal muscles; these symptoms can become progressively sharper, with patient having increasingly less control over voluntary movements and experiencing more involuntary ones.

- Eye movements become abnormal; eventually, patients cannot move their eyes.
- Other motor effects occur, such as increasing clumsiness, dysarthria, dysphagia, and ataxia.
- Cognitive symptoms start with confused thinking and progress to impaired communication, speech, and thinking processes.
- Emotional changes develop, including sleep and appetite disturbance, loss of energy, low self-esteem, increasing irritability, sudden anger, bipolar mood disorder, and suicidal tendencies; some Huntington's disease patients may have only these changes.
- In later stages of disease, complete immobility and muteness are seen.

▲ Health History:
Ask about a family history of or genetic markers for the disorder.

Chapter 27: Cranial Nerve Disorders

▽ ▽ ▽ ▽ ▽ ▽ ▽

INTRODUCTION

SEE TEXT PAGES

Disorders affecting the cranial nerves often result from another infection, trauma, disease, or disorder affecting the CNS. This chapter provides you with signs and symptoms and assessment instructions (particularly for the cranial nerves) for these disorders as well as for Tourette's syndrome, although it's not exclusively a sensory nerve deficit.

FACIAL PARALYSIS (BELL'S PALSY)

Although the exact cause of Bell's palsy, an idiopathic facial palsy, is unknown, a possible link may be compression of cranial nerve VII from inflammation due to viral or immune system disease. Eventually such compression can result in ischemia and degeneration of the nerve. Other possible causes include tumor or hemorrhage and local edema or infarct.

Unilateral paralysis may be complete or incomplete and may occur suddenly or develop over time (hours or days). Recovery may take days or months, often without the need for treatment. Ten percent of patients may experience permanent disfigurement.

NURSE ALERT

Because the patient may have difficulty closing the lid of the affected eye, suggest measures to protect the patient's cornea (for example, an eye patch and artifical tears).

SUPPORTING ASSESSMENT DATA

▲ Physical Findings:
- Pain around the ear
- Discomfort in the face, often around the eye; can progress to one-sided facial paralysis
- Diminished taste
- Diminished ability to close the eye and use the muscles around the mouth to smile, frown, or whistle

▲ Health History:
- First, diagnose by assessing the cranial nerves, taking a history, and evaluating signs and symptoms.

- Next, determine if a brain tumor or other mass is causing increased intracranial pressure that could affect the nerve.

TRIGEMINAL NEURALGIA (TIC DOULOUREUX)

Trigeminal neuralgia affects women more often than men with onset usually occurring after age 40. Causes of this disorder of the trigeminal nerve (cranial nerve V) include:
- Compression by blood vessel on the nerve
- Viral infection, particularly herpes zoster (atypical trigeminal neuralgia)
- Brain tumor or aneurysm (atypical trigeminal neuralgia)
- Multiple sclerosis (MS; atypical trigeminal neuralgia)

SUPPORTING ASSESSMENT DATA

▲ Physical Findings:
- Primary symptom is brief attacks of shooting, burning pain on one side of the face that cause the patient to grimace—hence, the tics.
- Attacks may be triggered by the presence of cold and by light touch or pressure on the affected areas (for example, lips, nose, chin, cheek).
- Attacks can last from a few seconds to a few minutes.

▲ Health History:
- It's important to rule out a severe underlying pathology, such as brain tumor or MS, which can cause atypical trigeminal neuralgia.

NURSE ALERT
A clue to the presence of tumor or MS is the age of the patient, who tends to be younger than those who typically have trigeminal neuralgia.

- Trigeminal neuralgia does not cause sensory loss in trigeminal distribution; atypical trigeminal neuralgia does.
- To assess for straightforward trigeminal neuralgia, test the suspected area with cold, pressure, or light touch to elicit the tic response.

MÉNIÈRE'S DISEASE

In Ménière's disease, which is associated with cranial nerve VIII, increased endolymphatic hydrops (fluid) is seen.

Causes include:
• Allergies
• Exposure to toxic substances
• Brain hemorrhage
• Localized ischemia

SUPPORTING ASSESSMENT DATA

▲ Physical Findings:
Many symptoms are similar to those seen with changes in the nerve responsible for hearing and equilibrium. The most common symptom is repeated episodes of vertigo. These symptoms may be accompanied by:
• Nausea and vomiting
• Tinnitus
• Nystagmus
• Hearing loss (temporary hearing loss can lead to partial or complete deafness)
• Feeling of fullness in the ear

▲ Health History:
• Examine the patient to rule out severe underlying disorders, such as brain hemorrhage or ischemia.
• Evaluate the patient's symptoms.
• Assess cranial nerve VIII.
• Use caloric testing to identify vestibular abnormalities.
• Perform audiometry to identify hearing loss and sensitivity to loud sounds.
• Keep in mind that occurrence of attacks ranges from weeks to years.
• Note that hearing is first affected in one ear and then advances to both ears.

GLOSSOPHARYNGEAL NEURALGIA
This disorder is typically caused by inflammation, compression, or injury to cranial nerve IX or by herpes zoster.

SUPPORTING ASSESSMENT DATA

▲ Physical Findings:
• Typical complaints include throat or ear pain; pain may be stimulated by any natural movements of the mouth and throat, such as laughing, yawning, swallowing, chewing, coughing, or blowing the nose.

▲ Health History:
• Ask about any exposure to herpes zoster.
• To diagnose, combine evaluation of symptoms with result of assessment of cranial nerve IX.

TOURETTE'S SYNDROME

This rare, hereditary disease is characterized by the following four criteria:

- Onset before age 21
- Multiple motor tics
- At least one vocal tic
- Lasts longer than 1 year

SUPPORTING ASSESSMENT DATA

▲ Physical Findings:

- Primary symptoms are motor, sensory, and phonic tics.
- Motor tics can include eye blinking, shrugs of the shoulder, jaw snaps, tooth clicking, and grimacing. They can advance to include biting, throwing, banging, and lewd gestures.
- Phonic tics include noises, such as hissing, barking, spitting, or sniffling. Complex phonic tics can manifest as actual, although inappropriate, statements, including the use of obscenities.
- Sensory tics are elusive, abnormal sensations of the skin, such as a tickle or pressure. Sensory tics are considered a warning for the more significant motor and phonic tics.
- Behavioral disturbances can include obsessive-compulsive disorder and attention deficit hyperactivity disorder.

▲ Health History:

- Observe for tics and behavioral disturbances by evaluating your patient's symptoms and observing the patient at work or in school.
- Take a thorough history to determine time of onset and progression and severity.
- Ask about a family history of the disease; additionally, obtain a developmental history and perform a neurologic assessment to eliminate other disorders.
- Use of stimulants can be connected to onset of the disorder; bronchodilators and decongestants can worsen tic symptoms.

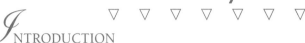 Chapter 28: Infections of the Central Nervous System

▽   ▽   ▽   ▽   ▽   ▽   ▽

INTRODUCTION

SEE TEXT PAGES

Infections of the CNS are highly dangerous and require immediate assessment and intervention to prevent irreparable damage or death. Conditions that can place the patient at risk for CNS infection include:

- Immune system compromise from underlying disorder, such as AIDS or lymphoma
- Use of immunosuppressive drugs
- Long-term debilitating conditions, such as renal failure
- Infections such as bacteremia
- Disruption of brain's protective system

BACTERIAL MENINGITIS

Bacterial meningitis is life-threatening; therefore, rapid assessment and diagnosis are crucial. Meningitis is most common in infants and children up to age 4 and in the elderly. The highest incidence of meningitis is in children up to age 1.

SUPPORTING ASSESSMENT DATA

The primary symptoms of meningeal infection are:
- Headache
- Stiff neck
- Fever

Other signs and symptoms include:
- Focal neurologic deficits
- Vomiting
- Nausea
- Photophobia
- Altered sensory functions
- Seizures
- Presence of Kernig's sign
- Presence of Brudzinski's sign

NURSE ALERT

Children under age 2 and the elderly may not experience the most obvious symptoms of meningitis. Young children may have only fever, poor nutritional intake, and a change in level of consciousness (LOC), such as lethargy or irritability. Elderly patients may not have a prominent fever or headache; their only signs and symptoms may be changes in mental status.

Serious potential complications of meningitis include increased intracranial pressure (ICP) because of inflammation, brain infarction, subdural fluid collection (particularly in infants), and hydrocephalus.

ASSESSMENT TECHNIQUES

Consider the patient's age because age influences whether meningitis is a prime concern. If age is a factor, determine patient's recent experiences to try to identify which organisms could have caused the meningitis.

THE CHILD

Assess infants for fontanelle bulging or increase of head circumference from subdural effusion (most commonly seen with *Haemophilus* meningitis).

NURSE ALERT

A lumbar puncture provides a definitive diagnosis of meningitis through cerebrospinal fluid (CSF) analysis. This procedure must be done immediately because the infection is life-threatening. This analysis can detect an increase in CSF pressure; confirm the presence of white blood cells, protein, and sugar; and identify bacteria that may be present.

VIRAL MENINGITIS

Also known as acute benign lymphocytic meningitis and acute aseptic meningitis, viral meningitis is not nearly as dangerous as bacterial meningitis. It usually occurs in small outbreaks and typically affects children.

SUPPORTING ASSESSMENT DATA

Like bacterial meningitis, viral meningitis includes these initial signs and symptoms:
- Fever
- Headache
- Stiff neck

Other signs and symptoms include:
- Elevated lymphocytes in the CSF; presence of lymphocytes in protective dura layers
- During acute stage, fever as high as 105° F (40.5° C); increased pulse and respiratory rates; level of consciousness that may decline from confusion to coma

ASSESSMENT TECHNIQUES

- Evaluate symptoms.
- Perform a general neurologic assessment.

BRAIN ABSCESS

Brain abscess, a focal infection in the brain, may be accompanied by meningitis. Although the disorder is rare, incidence is increasing because of the greater incidence of AIDS, penetrating head wounds, and I.V. drug use. Other causes and predisposing conditions include:

- Lung infections
- Endocarditis
- Chronic ear infection
- Mastoiditis
- Sinusitis
- Diabetes mellitus
- Bacteremia from a distant site of infection
- Recent infections or dental procedures
- Facial or scalp infections
- Immunocompromised status

The mortality rate for brain abscess is 30%, and the incidence of neurologic damage is 50%. A brain abscess is particularly dangerous because symptoms can appear slowly and increased ICP can develop. Furthermore, the necrotic material and pus that make up an abscess can destroy brain tissue.

SUPPORTING ASSESSMENT DATA

The most common signs and symptoms as a brain abscess progresses are fever and headache, either generalized or localized. Other signs and symptoms include nausea and vomiting, seizures, changes in mental status, and lethargy. Symptoms usually develop over the course of 2 weeks or less.

ASSESSMENT TECHNIQUES

- Monitor the patient's signs and symptoms.
- Take a history for any predisposing conditions.
- Perform a general neurologic assessment; note any localized neurologic defect on the physical examination.

IRAL ENCEPHALITIS (HERPES SIMPLEX ENCEPHALITIS)

In the United States, the most common cause of viral encephalitis, an inflammation of the brain, is the herpes simplex virus. Other causes include toxic substances and organisms such as bacteria, parasites, and fungi.

The most prevalent form of the disorder is herpes simplex encephalitis, caused by herpes simplex virus type 1. Although the virus is relatively benign in adults, usually causing oral lesions, it becomes serious when encephalitis occurs—causing death in almost one third of patients who receive treatment before coma and about three quarters of those who do not. Furthermore, many of those who survive herpes encephalitis have permanent neurologic defects.

The mechanism by which the virus enters the CNS is not known, but it is believed to spread along nerves into the brain. Commonly, herpes simplex type I infections affect the temporal lobes and can cause necrotic areas that may be hemorrhagic and associated with edema.

SUPPORTING ASSESSMENT DATA

The primary signs and symptoms, which develop and worsen over a few days, are:
- Fever
- Nausea and vomiting
- Headache
- Decreases in level of consciousness (confusion and stupor)
- Seizure
- Focal neurologic deficits
- Signs of increased ICP

ASSESSMENT TECHNIQUES

Although the signs and symptoms of viral encephalitis may indicate any number of disorders at first, it's important to consider this disorder because of its dangerous consequences. These guidelines can help with your assessment and diagnosis:
- Continually monitor the patient's condition and neurologic functioning.
- During history taking, ask about any history of or exposure to herpes simplex type 1 infection.

NURSE ALERT
A culture from a brain biopsy can confirm diagnosis.

HERPES ZOSTER (SHINGLES)

Shingles are caused by the chickenpox virus (varicella-zoster) that lies dormant in the dorsal root ganglia of peripheral nerves after an outbreak of chickenpox infection. The virus reactivates because of breakdown of the cells where it resides, causing it to multiply. The elderly and patients with compromised immune systems are most likely to develop the disease; incidence is extremely high among patients with AIDS.

SUPPORTING ASSESSMENT DATA

▼
▼
▼
▼
▼
▼
▼
▼
▼

- Initial symptoms include radicular pain and burning and itching.
- Several days later, as the virus continues to multiply, it reaches the vesicles at the nerve endings; vesicles grow larger and fill with pus before crusting over and eventually healing.
- Pain is present during and after recovery (called postherpetic neuralgia).
- In AIDS patients, look for the characteristic vesicular rash that is distributed over a dermatome and that seems to follow the pathway of the nerve.

ASSESSMENT TECHNIQUES

Evaluate symptoms and observe for the presence of vesicles and pain.

NURSE ALERT

Wear gloves when coming in contact with vesicles containing fluid.

AIDS

As a multisystem disorder, AIDS often affects the neurologic system. Neurologic conditions and other opportunistic diseases occur alone or concurrently in 30% of all AIDS patients. The types of disorders and processes that most frequently occur are:

- Primary infections: include atypical aseptic meningitis, encephalitis, and spinal vacuolar myelopathy and transverse myelitis (characterized by loss of posterior column sensation, spasticity, and presence of Babinski's reflex) as well as peripheral neuropathy.
- Opportunistic infections (viral and nonviral). Viral opportunistic infections include:

- herpes simplex encephalitis (usually fatal, causing progressive deficits)
- progressive multifocal leukoencephalopathy, (demyelinating, progressing to death with increasing
deficits such as blindness, aphasia, hemiparesis, ataxia, and diminished mental functioning)
- cytomegalovirus meningoencephalitis (usually causes blindness, with earlier symptoms of retinal detachment and visual field disturbances).
Nonviral opportunistic infections include:
- toxoplasmosis (abscess lesions in the brain, caused by *Toxoplasma gondii* protozoa and resulting in headache, confusion, seizures, paresis, and paralysis).
- cryptococcal meningitis (yeast infection characterized by fever, stiff neck, and headache).
• Tumors: CNS lymphomas can present with symptoms of memory loss, paralysis, aphasia, confusion, lethargy, and, in some cases, seizures. Diagnostic tests include a computed tomographic or magnetic resonance imaging scan, and a brain biopsy.
• Peripheral neuropathy: caused directly by human immunodeficiency virus (HIV) infection and nutritional deficits and presents as progressive, bilateral distal sensory loss.
• Dementia: can be caused by many of the infections and neuropathies seen with AIDS. AIDS dementia complex, however, is believed to be caused by a direct infection of the CNS by HIV. Signs and symptoms progress from cognitive and personality deficits to tremor, seizures, ataxia, hyperactive tendon reflexes, and, later, paraplegia and incontinence.

𝓛YME DISEASE

Lyme disease, a vector-borne infection, results from a deer tick (Ixodides) bite and causes a flulike illness that may involve the peripheral and central nervous systems. The disease is now endemic in certain regions of the United States: the Northeast (Massachusetts, Rhode Island, Connecticut, New York, New Jersey, Pennsylvania, Delaware, and Maryland), Midwest (Ohio, Illinois, Michigan, Iowa, Wisconsin, and Minnesota), Southeast (Georgia and North Carolina), and West (California, Nevada, Oregon, and Utah).

Lyme disease occurs in three stages. If it's not treated in the early stage, it can advance to cause neurologic disorders. About 15% of all patients develop neurologic complications.

SUPPORTING ASSESSMENT DATA

▼ First stage: Circular rash around the tick bite (the only
clear marker)
▼ Second stage:
▼ • Neck stiffness
▼ • Photophobia
▼ • Memory lapses
▼ • Arthritis
▼ • Headache
▼ • Facial palsy, spinal root syndromes, and other palsies
(indicates disease has advanced to chronic meningitis
and radiculitis)
▼ • Heart block
Third stage: Disease can advance to encephalitis and
demyelination, which can create signs and symptoms simi-
lar to those of multiple sclerosis, neurodegenerative
dementia, and neuropathies.

ASSESSMENT TECHNIQUES

• Ask whether the patient lives in or has recently traveled
to any of the states listed as high-risk areas.
• Ask whether the patient has recently hiked in woods or
fields or does any gardening
• Determine if the patient has any recent or past bites from
a tick.
• Look for a rash around the tick bite (in early stage).

CREUTZFELDT-JAKOB DISEASE

Creutzfeldt-Jakob disease—a relatively rare, subacute, progressive, and, ultimately, fatal disorder—is classified as a
spongiform encephalopathy (occurs in both humans and
animals). It is characterized by a long period of latency
between infection and the appearance of symptoms.

Subacute Creutzfeldt-Jakob disease is the most common
form of the disease, affecting more than 75% of those who
contract the illness. Patients usually die within 6 months of
the onset of symptoms. Chronic Creutzfeldt-Jakob disease
has symptoms similar to those of the subacute form, but
the disease may last at least 2 years. The rarest form, amyotrophic Creutzfeldt-Jakob disease, features fewer symptoms and can progress over many years. Transmission of
the disease is unclear, but evidence shows that a patient
has a high risk of infection if he comes into direct contact
with contaminated tissue or fluid.

SUPPORTING ASSESSMENT DATA
▼
▼
▼
▼
▼
▼
▼
▼
▼
▼
- Onset is sudden, with signs and symptoms similar to those of Alzheimer's disease: memory loss, language deficits, and personality and behavioral changes
- Myoclonic jerking
- Ataxia
- Nystagmus
- Dysarthria
- Hyperreflexia
- Spasticity
- Cortical blindness
- Seizures
- Sensory disturbances
- Coma and abnormal posturing (in last stage)

ASSESSMENT TECHNIQUES
- Evaluate the patient's signs and symptoms.
- Perform a general neurologic assessment.

GUILLAIN-BARRÉ SYNDROME

Guillain-Barré syndrome is an inflammatory disease of the peripheral nervous system that strikes suddenly, destroying the myelin sheath and thus preventing nerve impulses from passing. This loss of transmission causes paralysis, sensory loss, and dysfunction of the autonomic nervous system. Cognitive deficits are not usually present, although the patient can become extremely anxious and depressed because of the dramatic changes the disease creates. The disease ascends from the lower to the upper body, often requiring ventilator support, and usually resolves with time. Guillain-Barré syndrome occurs more often in males than in females.

The acute period of Guillain-Barré syndrome includes three phases:
- initial (lasts up to 3 weeks)
- plateau (lasts up to 2 weeks)
- recovery (can last up to 2 years)

Remyelination occurs in the recovery phase. Although no cure for Guillain-Barré syndrome is known, about 75% to 85% of affected patients recover.

SUPPORTING ASSESSMENT DATA
▼
▼
The signs and symptoms of Guillain-Barré syndrome worsen during the initial phase and stabilize during the plateau phase. These signs and symptoms include:
- Bilateral weakness in extremities

- Pain, tingling, and numbness in extremities
- Ataxia
- Facial weakness from cranial nerve effects
- Swallowing difficulty
- Increase in heart rate
- Increases or decreases in blood pressure
- Diminished breath and depth of respirations (ventilation may be necessary)
- Diminished or absent reflexes
- Possible heavy perspiration
- Intraocular muscle deficits

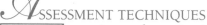

ASSESSMENT TECHNIQUES

- Assess the patient's signs and symptoms.
- Ask the patient if he has any difficulty swallowing or breathing.
- Perform a general neurologic assessment, particularly of the cranial nerves.

NURSE ALERT

Cranial nerve VII is one of the earliest nerves affected; as part of assessment, determine if the patient can voluntarily smile, close the eyes, or wrinkle the forehead.

RABIES

Rabies, a virus transmitted to humans through an animal bite, travels from the site of the bite along the axons to the spinal cord and brain and can include a long incubation period (from 10 days to 1 year). If no immediate treatment is given with rabies vaccine and rabies immune globulin, the disease is fatal.

SUPPORTING ASSESSMENT DATA

- Initial signs and symptoms occur during the subacute phase, which lasts for 3 to 4 days, and include headache, hyperexcitability, and changes in personality.
- Later signs and symptoms: facial spasms, dysphagia, and pharyngeal muscle spasms (the latter two cause drooling and inability to swallow water, which is seen as frothing at the mouth and so-called hydrophobia); eventually, seizures and coma.

ASSESSMENT TECHNIQUES

- Ask whether the patient was recently bitten by an animal and, if so, how it happened. Also ask if the animal exhibited any unusual behavior; note that wild animals often do not show any signs of rabies.
- Ask whether the patient recently explored any caves; bat

feces are aerosolized and may contain the rabies virus, which can be inhaled.

- For the patient who was bitten, ask if the bite was from a domestic animal (for example, a dog or cat). Domestic animals must be impounded, checked for immunization status, and observed for 10 days before patient is immunized. If the domestic animal cannot be found, treatment should be administered immediately.
- The only way to confirm rabies is by trapping the animal and testing it for characteristic cells (cytoplasmic inclusion or Negri body).
- For all wild animal bites, regardless of whether the animal is found, prophylaxis is necessary immediately after the bite occurs (and before symptoms appear) with a series of immunizations and rabies immune globulin.

$\mathcal{S}$UGGESTED READINGS

Chokroverty, Sudhansu, ed. *Movement Disorders.* Lyons, NJ: PMA Publishing Corp., 1990.

Cook, Stuart D., ed. *Handbook of Multiple Sclerosis.* New York: Marcel Dekker, Inc., 1990.

Geary, Siobhan M. "Nursing Management of Cranial Nerve Dysfunction." *Journal of Neuroscience Nursing* 27 (April 1995): 102–108.

Gillespie, Marjorie M. "Tremor." *Journal of Neuroscience Nursing* 23 (June 1991): 170–174.

Habermann-Little, Barbara. "An Analysis of the Prevalence and Etiology of Depression with Parkinson's Disease." *Journal of Neuroscience Nursing* 23 (June 1991): 165–169.

Jankovis, Joseph, and Eduardo Tolosa. *Parkinson's Disease and Movement Disorders.* 2nd ed. Baltimore: William & Wilkins, 1993.

Schlossberg, David, ed. *Infections of the Nervous System.* New York: Springer-Verlag, 1990.

Skodal Wilson, Holly. "Nursing the Mind Easing Life for the Alzheimer's Patient." *RN* 53 (December 1990): 24–28.

Tariot, Pierre N. "Alzheimer Disease: An Overview." *Alzheimer Disease and Associated Disorders* 8 (Supp. 2, 1994): S4–S11.

INDEX

ORDER OTHER TITLES IN THIS SERIES!

INSTANT NURSING ASSESSMENT:

▲ Cardiovascular	0-8273-7102-0
▲ Respiratory	0-8273-7099-7
▲ Neurologic	0-8273-7103-9
▲ Women's Health	0-8273-7100-4
▲ Gerontologic	0-8273-7101-2
▲ Mental Health	0-8273-7104-7
▲ Pediatric	0-8273-7098-9

RAPID NURSING INTERVENTIONS

▲ Cardiovascular	0-8273-7105-5
▲ Respiratory	0-8273-7095-4
▲ Neurologic	0-8273-7093-8
▲ Women's Health	0-8273-7092-X
▲ Gerontologic	0-8273-7094-6
▲ Mental Health	0-8273-7096-2
▲ Pediatric	0-8273-7097-0

- - - - - - - - - - - - - - - ✂ (cut here) - - - - - - - - - - - - - - -

GET "INSTANT" EXPERIENCE!

QTY.	TITLE / ISBN	PRICE	TOTAL
		19.95	
		19.95	
		19.95	
		19.95	
		19.95	
		19.95	
		SUBTOTAL	
		STATE OR LOCAL TAXES	
		TOTAL	

Payment Information
☐ A Check is Enclosed
☐ Charge my ☐ VISA ☐ Mastercard CARD #_____

NAME _____
SCHOOL/INSTITUTION _____
STREET ADDRESS _____
CITY/STATE/ZIP _____
HOME PHONE _____
OFFICE PHONE _____

MAIL OR FAX COMPLETED FORM TO:
Delmar Publishers • P.O. Box 15015 • Albany, NY 12212-5015

IN A HURRY TO ORDER? FAX: 1-518-464-0301
OR CALL TOLL-FREE 1-800-347-7707